ENGAGING THE INTERSECTION OF HOUSING AND HEALTH

T0385658

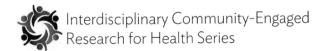 Interdisciplinary Community-Engaged
Research for Health Series

The *Interdisciplinary Community-Engaged Research for Health* series aims to bridge the gap between researchers and practitioners to facilitate the development of collaborative, equitable research and action. The reality of persistent health disparities and structural inequalities highlights the need for new strategies that are social justice-driven. Traditionally, efforts have tended to be institution-based, "expert"-focused, and silo-specific. To promote health equity, diverse stakeholders with different types of expertise need to work together to solve real-world problems. This series publishes books that recognize the importance of diverse collaboration and equip readers from a variety of backgrounds with the tools and vision to center community voice in research for action.

Series Editors:

Farrah Jacquez
University of Cincinnati

Lina Svedin
University of Utah

Advisory Board:

Sherrie Flynt Wallington
George Washington University

Jennifer Malat
University of Cincinnati

Kristin Kalsem
University of Cincinnati

Kathleen Thiede Call
University of Minnesota

Andriana Abariotes
University of Minnesota

ENGAGING THE INTERSECTION OF HOUSING AND HEALTH

Interdisciplinary Community-Engaged Research for Health Series

Volume 3

Edited by Mina Silberberg

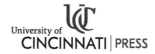

University of
CINCINNATI | PRESS

About the University of Cincinnati Press

The University of Cincinnati Press is committed to publishing rigorous, peer-reviewed, leading scholarship accessibly to stimulate dialog among the academy, public intellectuals and lay practitioners. The Press endeavors to erase disciplinary boundaries in order to cast fresh light on common problems in our global community. Building on the university's long-standing tradition of social responsibility to the citizens of Cincinnati, state of Ohio, and the world, the press publishes books on topics that expose and resolve disparities at every level of society and have local, national and global impact.

The University of Cincinnati Press, Cincinnati 45221
Copyright © 2022

ISBN 978-1-947602-72-4 (paperback)
ISBN 978-1-947602-74-8 (e-book, PDF)
ISBN 978-1-947602-73-1 (e-book, EPUB)

Silberberg, Mina (Mina R.), editor.
Engaging the intersection of housing and health / edited by Mina Silberberg.
Cincinnati : The University of Cincinnati Press, 2022. |
   Series: Interdisciplinary community-engaged research for health ; volume 3 | Includes bibliographical references and index.
LCCN 2020055852 | ISBN 9781947602724 (paperback) | ISBN 9781947602731 (epub) | ISBN 9781947602748 (pdf)
LCSH: Housing and health—United States. | Housing policy—United States. | Medical policy—United States. | Social policy—Research—Methodology.
LCC RA770 .E55 2021 | DDC 362.10973—dc23
LC record available at https://lccn.loc.gov/2020055852

Designed and produced for UC Press by Jennifer Flint
Typeset in Granjon LT Std
Printed in the United States of America
First Printing

Contents

ENGAGING THE INTERSECTION OF HOUSING AND HEALTH

Chapter 1

Engaging the Intersection of Housing and Health

Changing Research to Change Policy

Mina Silberberg

Researchers often hope that their work will inform social change. The questions that motivate us to pursue research careers in the first place often stem from observations about gaps between the world as we wish it to be and the world as it is, accompanied by a deep curiosity about how it might be made different. If research is to inform social change, however, we must first change some aspects of the way in which research is done. This book offers case studies of research that is interdisciplinary, community-engaged, and intentionally designed for translation into practice.[1] In this introductory chapter I will outline the rationale for this approach to research, contextualizing the cases that follow.

---

1. We will not in this book address distinctions among the terms "multidisciplinary," "interdisciplinary," and "transdisciplinary" (see, e.g., Choi and Pak, 2006). Rather, we will use the term "interdisciplinary" because it appears in the name of the fellowship program that generated this volume (RWJF, n.d.). In this context, we understand the term to encompass a variety of ways in which practitioners and paradigms from different fields can be brought together.

The Need for Interdisciplinary, Stakeholder-Engaged, Translational Research

A growing body of evidence demonstrates that diverse sectors like health, housing, and education and academic disciplines like biology and sociology are intertwined. In the field of population health, in particular, there is now consensus that the biggest drivers of health are not medical care, health education, and physiology, but rather psychosocial factors, socioeconomic conditions, and the physical environment (Frieden, 2010). Health, in turn, can be a driver of other social realities, such as labor productivity and educational attainment (Mitchell & Bates, 2011; Murray et al., 2007). Given these relationships, improved health cannot be achieved through the expertise and efforts of the health sector alone, nor are education issues solely the province of educators. The fact that health is shaped by social conditions is not new; it is evident across societies and across time (Link & Phelan, 1995). However, this intersection—particularly the effects of "social drivers of health"—is now part of the discourse of mainstream institutions from the U.S. Office of Disease Prevention and Health Promotion (ODPHP, n.d.) to the World Health Organization.

There are numerous ways in which housing and health are intertwined. This intertwining—which is the focus of this volume—is lived daily by the children whose asthma is exacerbated by mold in their homes, the adults whose chronic mental illness increases their risk for homelessness and whose homelessness worsens their mental *and* physical health, the seniors whose home environment heightens their risk of falls, and the families who must choose between paying for housing and paying for healthcare.

While our understanding of the intersections among diverse subjects has grown, fields of study and practice have become increasingly specialized and numerous (Law & Kim, 2005). Of particular note for the study and practice of health improvement is the history of public health and medicine in the United States; once a common endeavor, they became separate fields in the twentieth century (Brandt & Gardner, 2000). If we are to address our social needs, we must escape the silos that arise with the proliferation of disciplines. In 2003, Elias Zerhouni, then director of the National Institutes of Health (NIH), made this point when he wrote that the specialization and decentralization that had benefited the work of NIH in the past needed to be supplemented by collaboration across disciplines. "Solving the puzzle of complex diseases," he noted, "from obesity to cancer, will require a holistic understanding of the interplay between factors such as genetics, diet, infectious agents, environment, behavior, and social structures" (Zerhouni, 2003, p. 64).

Zerhouni noted that, in addition to working across disciplines, we need to address barriers to the "translation" of research into practice. The mismatch between the siloed nature of much research and the interdisciplinary nature of real-world problems is only one such barrier. Although Zerhouni was particularly concerned with the translation of research into medical practice (Zerhouni, 2006), the importance of social and environmental drivers of health necessitates that we also pursue the translation of knowledge about housing, education, the environment, and so on into changes in policy.

There are many barriers to the translation of research into practice. They include lack of trust between researchers and practitioners, a lack of researcher training for communication with nonspecialists, differing priorities, mismatched timelines for the production of knowledge (with the practice field generally requiring faster results), the failure of researchers to appreciate the importance of context in an intervention's success, and their lack of appreciation for the insights gained from lived experience (Wallerstein & Duran, 2010). Moreover, the costs accruing to specific stakeholders from change can be a powerful incentive for those stakeholders to maintain the status quo. The tobacco industry, for example, has worked hard to blunt policy changes designed to reduce use of their product (Smith, Savell, & Gilmore, 2013). Even the incentives for change in the nonprofit sector are a topic of significant debate (Larsen, 2016). Arguably, then, all translation-oriented research requires an understanding of the sociopolitical dynamics of the relevant field, making it interdisciplinary by definition. Finally, as Ogilvie and colleagues (2009) have argued, the linear model of knowledge transfer from scientists to clinical practice, which, in this author's view, may not even be effective in the strictly medical realm, is clearly not effective for addressing population health problems that are driven by diverse factors with causal pathways at the policy, systems, societal, *and* individual levels. For example, they note, translating knowledge about sodium into clinical practice will have limited impact when most salt is not added by the consumer but comes from processed foods. Advising parents to vaccinate children will not be effective when researchers refuse to try to understand parents' fears that vaccination is linked to autism.

Translation of research to practice and movement from practice to population health improvement, therefore, are not easy tasks but require proactive attention and investment to create the necessary preconditions and dynamics for effective translation to take place. One important strategy for facilitating translation is stakeholder engagement in research. Stakeholders include those directly affected by an issue, that is, in the case of health, those whose health is at stake; actors who are responsible for or will sustain costs or benefits from policy, systems, or practice change;

or change advocates. In the health field, involvement of the community whose health will be directly affected is often referred to as community engagement, defined by the Centers for Disease Control and Prevention (CDC) as "the process of working collaboratively with and through groups of people affiliated by geographic proximity, special interest, or similar situations to address issues affecting the well-being of those people" (CDC, 2011). The term "community engagement" is also often used to refer to the broader array of stakeholder-engaged approaches; in this context, the community can be, for example, collaborators from outside of the research institution. In this volume, in order to align with a number of current initiatives, it is this broader use of the term "community engagement" (i.e., interchangeable with stakeholder engagement) that we will employ. However, we do so with the recognition that the benefits and challenges of engaging different types of stakeholders vary by type of stakeholder (as well as from study to study within stakeholder types) and that this variation must be critically assessed.

Wallerstein and Duran (2010) note that community-based participatory research (CBPR)—a particular approach to community engagement—facilitates research translation by enhancing trust between researchers and the community, creating hybrid knowledge informed by both research and lived realities, and developing bidirectional learning. They further note that CBPR facilitates translation by promoting the sharing of resources, collective decision-making, a focus on outcomes beneficial to the community, adaptation of interventions to specific contexts, and approaches to change that are sustainable within existing structures. The same argument can be made for stakeholder-engaged research more generally. Which stakeholders should be engaged in a specific study depends on the nature of the field of inquiry, the skills and expertise of the researchers and potential partners, and the study's aims.

The crucial point is that stakeholder engagement can be a powerful tool for translation.

As with the importance of social drivers of health, the concept of stakeholder-engaged research is not new. In the first half of the twentieth century, Kurt Lewin advanced "action research," promoting stakeholder engagement for practical problem-solving (Wallerstein & Duran, 2017), although stakeholder-engaged research undoubtedly predates even this formal recognition. As is also the case with social drivers of health, what is new is mainstream recognition of the potential importance of this approach (CDC, 2011), including funding support from institutions like the NIH.

The Need to Develop Our Capacity for Translation-Oriented Research

The interdisciplinary, community-engaged, and translational research just described is significantly different from the research most commonly supported by and conducted within academic institutions. Academic training, departmental structures, and promotion criteria and timelines encourage researchers to delve deeply into narrow areas of expertise and to focus their time and efforts on dissemination to other researchers in their fields through peer-reviewed publication rather than on the time-consuming work of forging the relationships that undergird interdisciplinary collaboration and stakeholder engagement or on dissemination to and translation for the practice community (Marrero et al., 2013). Academic training prepares researchers to succeed in this institutional context.

As a result, conducting research that is interdisciplinary, community-engaged, and translation-oriented requires attitudes, skills, and behaviors that are not taught in most research training programs and can even be disincentivized by academic structures. In recognition of the need to develop a new type of research capacity, the Robert Wood Johnson Foundation (RWJF) launched the Interdisciplinary Research Leaders (IRL) Fellowship Program in 2016. This program awards funding to teams comprising two researchers and one community partner. As described by RWJF, IRL is "a leadership development opportunity for teams of researchers and community partners, including community organizers and advocates. These teams use the power of applied research—informing and supporting critical work being done in communities—to accelerate the work and advance health and equity" (RJWF, n.d.).

In addition to carrying out an interdisciplinary, community-engaged project with a translation orientation, IRL fellows receive training in engaging stakeholders; applying research and data to program and policy design and operations; integrating equity, cultures of health, and other key concepts into their work; advocating for systemic change to improve health and health equity; and building public will to address health-related issues.

The goal of this volume and the others in the Interdisciplinary Community-Engaged Research for Health series is to expand the learning fostered by the IRL program and similar initiatives by disseminating the experiences and lessons of what we will term here "interdisciplinary community-engaged research" or ICEnR. This volume includes case studies of four IRL teams and two other collaborations addressing the nexus of housing and health. Our hope is that this content will motivate both researchers and community members to collaborate on translation-oriented research, provide guidance for this work, and raise important questions about how to maximize its benefits.

The Content of This Volume

This introduction is followed by six case studies of ICEnR. The first case, by George Mugoya, Billy Kirkpatrick, Pamela Payne Foster, Shameka Cody, and Safiya George, describes a study designed to improve the health of people living with HIV and AIDS in rural Alabama. Mugoya and George—both faculty at the University of Alabama at the time—and Kirkpatrick, chief executive officer of Five Horizons Health Services, initiated their partnership in response to challenges to prevention and treatment of HIV/AIDS associated with lack of access to housing, social stigma, inadequate transportation, and a generalized pattern of racial and socioeconomic disparities in health and access to resources. As the chapter describes, the partnership expanded to include additional research faculty and staff, as well as peer leaders from among the population served by Five Horizons. The case study demonstrates the benefits of this partnership for addressing the complex array of challenges faced by individuals living with HIV and AIDS, especially in rural areas. An intriguing aspect of this case study is its description of how the team identified and learned how to take advantage of the unique talents of each of its members. The project's training of peer leaders was also an important component of its approach to engaging and benefiting the community.

The second case study, by Leslie Taylor-Grover and Revathi Hines, provides an extensive history of racism, residential segregation, and associated trauma in Baton Rouge, Louisiana. Informed by this history and research on the sequelae of historical trauma, the authors—both faculty at Southern University—began a series of "Community Conversations" in collaboration with nonprofit organizations Assisi House and Resilient Baton Rouge. The goal of these conversations was to learn from the city's residents about the interaction between housing and health in both everyday life and after natural disasters. The authors also interviewed policymakers and found that when discussed in the community context, "notions of health took on a completely different connotation that policymakers imagined" (chapter 3, p. 50). This finding demonstrates the importance of amplifying the voices of community members, especially those whose health is at stake. The authors note both the benefits and challenges of this work, highlighting the difficulty they encountered in engaging city residents most affected by racism and trauma.

While the first two case studies describe research partnerships with wide-ranging agendas, the third describes a study designed to inform the regulatory framework associated with a specific policy decision: the use of Medicaid funding for case management to help individuals who are institutionalized or homeless obtain and maintain community-based housing. Researchers Mina Silberberg and Donna Biederman from Duke University partnered with Emily Carmody of the North Carolina Coalition to End Homelessness to address questions about regulatory design initially posed by Carmody. The authors argue that, while community engagement is not often solicited in regulatory research, this approach has great benefits, as does the inclusion on the research team of an advocate for homeless services; among the benefits of engagement of this advocate was the way in which it facilitated wider community engagement. The case study illustrates the strengths of this approach, its challenges, and strategies for addressing these challenges.

The next case study, by Christina Stacy and Joseph Schilling of the Urban Institute and Steven Barlow of Neighborhood Preservation Inc., Memphis, describes their collaboration on a health impact assessment of housing code enforcement policies and programs. Health impact assessment—developed in recognition of the importance of social and environmental drivers of health—is used to estimate the health implications of policy and program options, just as environmental impact assessment facilitates consideration of the environmental impact of policy and programmatic choices. The case study demonstrates how health impact assessments can serve as a vehicle for facilitating cross-sector collaboration at the intersection of housing and public health, the importance of stakeholder engagement for research translation, and the relationship between housing code enforcement and health.

The chapter by Donna Biederman and her colleagues describes a long-term, multifaceted collaboration between the Duke University School of Nursing (DUSON) and the Durham (NC) Housing Authority (DHA) that is helping to improve the quality of life for DHA residents, supporting the work of the DHA, enhancing the education of DUSON students, and facilitating research by the school's faculty. The chapter illustrates how a collaboration can evolve over time from its initial focus to encompass a variety of shared activities that are mutually beneficial for the partners. The case also shows that this longevity and expansion require an investment on the part of faculty in building relationships in the community, including a commitment to flexibility, transparency, and showing up to events that matter to your partners.

In their case study, Lina Svedin and Jesus Valero of the University of Utah describe how they responded to a request by the Division of Housing and Community Development of the Utah Department of Workforce Services to provide research support to the development of the state's strategic plan on homelessness. They and their team accomplished this task in less than three-and-a-half months—truly impressive when you consider what they describe as "the snail-like speed with which administrative and research approval processes churn in academia" (chapter 7, page 143) and the usual length of an academic research project. The conflict between academic and policymaker timelines is one of the key challenges to the translation of research into policy. Svedin and Valero's description of how they met the deadline they were given—while still remaining engaged with the state and making sure that their research represented multiple stakeholder voices—offers hope and a roadmap for meeting this and other challenges of translational research.

The last chapter of this volume provides critical reflections on the case studies we have included. It addresses the ways in which these cases illustrate the benefits of ICEnR, the challenges of this work, and the strategies and infrastructure that can support its success. The concluding chapter also raises questions for further study. The fundamental rationale behind the approach described in this volume is that it offers the insight to be gained by bringing together diverse skills and perspectives. In that spirit, we invite readers to draw their own conclusions and frame their own questions based on what is presented here.

References

Brandt, A., & Gardner, M. (2000). Antagonism and accommodation: Interpreting the relationship between public health and medicine in the United States during the 20th century. *American Journal of Public Health, 90*(5), 707–715. https://doi.org/10.2105/AJPH.90.5.707

Centers for Disease Control and Prevention (CDC). (2011). *Principles of community engagement* (2nd ed.). Washington, DC: Department of Health and Human Services.

Choi, B.C.K., & Pak, A.W.P. (2006). Multidisciplinarity, interdisciplinarity, and transdisciplinarity in health research, services, education, and policy: Definitions, objectives, and evidence of effectiveness. *Clinical and Investigative Medicine/ Médecine Clinique et Experimentale, 29*(6), 351.

Frieden, T. R. (2010). A framework for public health action: The health impact pyramid. *American Journal of Public Health, 100*(4), 590–595. https://doi.org/10.2105/AJPH.2009.185652

Larsen, P. (2016). The good, the ugly, and the Dirty Harrys of conservation: Rethinking the anthropology of conservation NGOs. *Conservation and Society, 14*(1), 21.

Law, M., & Kim, S. (2005). Specialization and regulation: The rise of professionals and the emergence of occupational licensing regulation. *Journal of Economic History, 65*(3), 723–756. https://doi.org/10.1017/S0022050705000264

Link, B. G., & Phelan, J. (1995). Social conditions as fundamental causes of disease. *Journal of Health and Social Behavior,* Spec. no., 80.

Marrero, D. G., Hardwick, E. J., Staten, L. K., Savaiano, D. A., Odell, J. D., Comer, K. F., & Saha, C. (2013). Promotion and tenure for community-engaged research: An examination of promotion and tenure support for community-engaged research at three universities collaborating through a clinical and translational science award. *Clinical and Translational Science, 6*(3), 204–208. https://doi.org/10.1111/cts.12061

Mitchell, R. J., & Bates, P. (2011). Measuring health-related productivity loss. *Population Health Management, 14*(2), 93–98. https://doi.org/10.1089/pop.2010.0014

Murray, N. G., Low, B. J., Hollis, C., Cross, A. W., & Davis, S. M. (2007). Coordinated school health programs and academic achievement: A systematic review of the literature. *Journal of School Health, 77*(9), 589–600.

Office of Disease Prevention and Health Promotion (ODPHP). (n.d.). *Social determinants of health.* Retrieved May 29, 2021, from https://www.healthypeople.gov/2020/topics-objectives/topic/social-determinants-of-health

Ogilvie, D., Craig, P., Griffin, S., Macintyre, S., & Wareham, N. J. (2009). A translational framework for public health research. *BMC Public Health, 9*,116.

Robert Wood Johnson Foundation (RWJF). (n.d.). *Interdisciplinary research leaders.* Retrieved June 11, 2019, from https://interdisciplinaryresearch-leaders.org/about-the-program/

Smith, K. E., Savell, E., & Gilmore, A. B. (2013). What is known about tobacco industry efforts to influence tobacco tax? A systematic review of empirical studies. *Tobacco Control, 22*, e1.

Wallerstein, N., & Duran, B. (2010). Community-based participatory research contributions to intervention research: The intersection of science and practice to improve health equity. *American Journal of Public Health, 100*(Suppl. 1), S40–S46. https://doi.org/10.2105/AJPH.2009.184036

Wallerstein, N., & Duran, B. (2017). Theoretical, historical, and practice roots of CBPR. In N. Wallerstein, B. Duran, J. G. Oetzel, & M. Minkler (Eds.), *Community-based participatory research for health: Advancing social and health equity* (3rd ed.) (17–30). Jossey-Bass.

Zerhouni, E. (2003). Medicine: The NIH roadmap. *Science, 302*(5642), 63–72. https://doi.org/10.1126/science.1091867

Zerhouni, E. A. (2006). Clinical research at a crossroads. *Journal of Investigative Medicine, 54*(4), 171.

Chapter 2

Combating HIV Stigma in Rural Alabama

*Importance of Peer Leadership, Interdisciplinary Research,
and Community Collaboration*

George C. T. Mugoya, Billy Kirkpatrick, Pamela Payne-Foster, Shameka Cody,
and Safiya George

*Five Horizons, an Alabama AIDS service organization, recognizes that housing
is essential to the well-being of people living with HIV/AIDS (PLWHA), and
includes affordable housing as an integral requirement for its clientele. The
agency also recognizes that the intersection of housing and health extends to the
issue of* where *one is housed. In rural Alabama, stigma, overt and structural
racism, and conservative societal values isolate PLWHA. Moreover, living
in a rural community presents challenges to accessing medical care. Finally,
research indicates that PLWHA residing in the rural South are more likely
than the general population to experience depression and anxiety and to have
a history of substance abuse, yet they are less likely to have access to treatment
for these needs. It is in response to these problems that our team of interdisciplinary researchers, community leaders (including the chief executive officer
of Five Horizons), and peer leaders came together to find ways to reduce HIV-
related stigma, address substance abuse and mental health issues for PLWHA,
and improve treatment adherence. The research, driven by a deep personal and
professional commitment to health equity in West Alabama, is anchored in the*

belief that access to healthcare and the ability to influence health policy are of paramount importance. This chapter highlights the experiences and lessons learned in this collaborative endeavor aimed at improving health outcomes among PLWHA in West Alabama. The strength of the partnerships developed through the process of this community-engaged research has been a major asset when confronted with challenges. For instance, literature has documented that despite being disproportionately affected by HIV/AIDS in the United States, minorities continue to be underrepresented in HIV/AIDS clinical trials. As a result of our partnerships with the community and the integral role of peer leaders in our work, participation in the projects we have been involved in has been excellent. Partnership has also enabled us to come up with community-driven and evidence-based solutions, for example, conducting counseling via telehealth in a manner that is acceptable to clients, assures confidentiality, and is founded on an evidence-based theoretical framework.

Numerous regional disparities exist in rates of HIV infection, people living with HIV/AIDS (PLWHA), AIDS-related deaths, and HIV outcomes in the United States. Specifically, the southern United States has reported disproportionately high HIV diagnosis and mortality rates compared to other U.S. regions (CDC, 2014; Reif et al., 2016). Because the prevalence and sequelae of chronic conditions such as HIV/AIDS often have related sociocultural risk factors (Payne-Foster et al., 2018), creating and fostering partnerships among all community stakeholders is vital to achieving optimal health outcomes. This is especially true when such individuals come from vulnerable populations. This chapter highlights a collaboration that brought together community leaders, peers, and interdisciplinary researchers, including the chapter authors. We describe the process of forming the collaboration and highlights of our successes.

Background

HIV/AIDS Prevalence and Issues Related to Prevention and Treatment

In 2013, approximately 40 percent of individuals diagnosed with HIV resided in the Deep South (comprising Alabama, Florida, Georgia, Louisiana, Mississippi, North Carolina, South Carolina, Tennessee, and Texas), while this region accounted for only 28 percent of the U.S. population (Reif et al., 2017). During the same period, the Deep South also faced the highest death rates among individuals diagnosed with HIV (Reif et al., 2017).

Racial disparities have also been reported in HIV infection and deaths. Compared to other racial/ethnic groups, African Americans account for a higher proportion of all stages of HIV disease—from new infections to deaths. These disparities are especially pronounced in the rural Southeast (Adimora et al., 2003). For example, in Alabama—the setting for the current study—the latest data from the Alabama Department of Public Health (ADPH) indicated that African Americans made up approximately 26.8 percent of the population in the state yet accounted for 71 percent of new HIV diagnoses and 64 percent of all PLWHA (ADPH, 2019).

Some of the factors that have been associated with these disparities, especially among African Americans in the rural South, include differential drug use due to isolation, which leads to increased HIV risk and stigma. Research indicates that PLWHA are more likely than those in the general population to experience depression and anxiety and to have a history of substance abuse, yet they are less likely to have access to treatment, especially in the rural South (CDC, 2014; Horstmann et al., 2010). HIV-related stigma has also been identified as one of the main factors in the rural South associated with increasing rates of HIV infections and their negative consequences. Indeed, extant literature indicates that societal stigma associated with race and ethnicity contributes to general disparities in mental and physical health (Williams & Mohammed, 2009) and healthcare (Nelson, 2002). Racial minorities "living with HIV often possess other stigmas beyond their race/ethnicity, including HIV itself and related stigmas such as sexual minority orientation, transgender identity or expression, illicit drug use, sex work, incarceration, and immigration" (Earnshaw et al., 2013, p. 227).

Differences in sexual networks between African Americans and White people have also been hypothesized as connected to a potential disparity observed in HIV infections in the rural South. Adimora and colleagues, in a study involving African American men and women who had been reported to the North Carolina HIV/Sexually Transmitted Disease Prevention and Care Section within the preceding six months because of HIV infection found that a majority reported having participated in concurrent partnerships and also believed that their partners had had sexual relationships with others during their relationship with the respondents (Adimora et al., 2003).

Treatment of PLWHA with highly active antiretroviral therapy (HAART), which generally decreases viral loads to undetectable levels if utilized consistently, has been a cornerstone in the treatment of HIV. PLWHA who are virally suppressed have significantly lower HIV transmission rates than PLWHA not engaged in care (Lichtenstein, 2007). However, despite significant scale-up of HIV treatment across the globe, the overall effectiveness of HIV treatment is severely undermined by attrition of PLWHA across the HIV care continuum (Reif et al., 2017). In the United States, linkage to and retention in care among PLWHA has generally been worse among younger persons, females, and racial/ethnic minorities (Adimora et al., 2003; CDC, 2012; Magnus et al., 2010;

Mugavero et al., 2013). For example, only 28 percent of African Americans infected with HIV are virally suppressed. Several factors—including HIV stigma, lack of health insurance, substance abuse, and unmet needs for supportive services including housing, case management, mental health, and substance abuse services—have been consistently associated with poor or inconsistent HIV care engagement (Mugavero et al., 2013).

HIV Stigma among PLWHA in Rural South

HIV-related stigma, defined as the shame or disgrace attached to the HIV diagnosis and expressed through negative social reactions toward people infected with HIV, is a detriment to HIV treatment and prevention. Stigma is associated with emotional distress, treatment delays, and poor health outcomes for a number of diseases. The adverse psychosocial effects of stigma include guilt, embarrassment, isolation, fear, and denial following a diagnosis, meaning that PLWHA are concerned about both the social and physical impact of the disease on their lives. The internalization of either anticipated or experienced stigma among PLWHA creates negative self-perceptions, feelings of inferiority, guilt, and concerns about disclosure (Foster, 2007; Herek, 1999). This leads to limited disclosure (Mugavero et al., 2013), self-isolation (Herek, Capatanio, & Widaman, 2002), decreased access to healthcare services, and decreased medication adherence (Emlet, 2005).

Culturally conservative views regarding HIV transmission (Horstmann et al., 2010) have been identified as one of the main sources of HIV stigma. Indeed, stigma surrounding HIV infection in the rural South is closely linked to assumptions that those who contract HIV do so through activity considered morally "deviant," particularly sexual activity and injection drug use (Mugavero et al., 2013).

Alabama sits in the Deep South, an area also referred to as the "Bible Belt" due to the strong connections that residents have with religion (Mahajan et al., 2008). Closely related are traditional beliefs about gender/ sexuality that have been linked with greater HIV-related stigma (Nunn et al., 2013; Warf & Winsberg, 2008); however, religious affiliation is not always a significant predictor of increased HIV-related stigma, perhaps due to a shift in church teachings in some cases (Nunn et al., 2013; Warf & Winsberg, 2008).

Interventions aimed at reducing HIV stigma among church leaders and members throughout the United States (in the Midwest and California) show promise; most studies, however, focus on urban African American and Latino populations (Berkley-Patton et al., 2013; Foster, Thomas, & Lewis, 2016). Researchers have begun to conduct studies in rural areas to better characterize the effect of faith-based organizations on HIV stigma against persons living with HIV, HIV prevention, and HIV research engagement. Payne-Foster and colleagues (2018), in surveying twenty-four African American PLWHA, found that participants felt most stigmatized by churches (Smith, Simmons, & Mayer, 2005). Of significance is a pilot study implemented by Payne-Foster and colleagues (2018) that developed a faith-based, anti-stigma intervention with twelve African American churches in rural Alabama. Measuring levels of HIV-related stigma held by 199 adults who participated in the intervention (individual-level) and their perception of stigma among other congregants (congregational-level), results indicated those who participated in the anti-stigma intervention reported a significant reduction in individual-level stigma compared to the control group (Lindley, Coleman, & Gaddist, 2010). Studies have also examined rural pastors in Alabama in HIV prevention activities and have identified barriers to engagement as well as factors predicting which pastors were most likely to engage. Factors encouraging pastor engagement included a spouse who worked in a health-related field, being previously engaged in social justice work, and/or having reverse migrated from metropolitan areas to the South. The cumulative effect of these findings might provide clues on best practices for enlisting African American rural southern pastors in faith-based HIV prevention, HIV stigma awareness, and HIV research (Foster, Thomas, & Lewis, 2016).

Community-Based Partnership and Engagement

Given that "chronic conditions are rooted not only in physiological processes, but also in sociocultural [factors]" (Payne-Foster et al., 2018), it is vital to involve all community stakeholders as partners if we are to achieve optimal health outcomes for individuals with chronic illness, especially in vulnerable populations (Payne-Foster et al., 2018; Plumb et al., 2012). Such collaboration becomes even more essential for a chronic illness as highly stigmatized as HIV/AIDS. Establishing such partnerships, however, are challenging. Past research indicates minority populations are less likely to participate in research projects; for example, African Americans diagnosed with HIV/AIDS are less likely to be enrolled in research projects when compared to national averages (El-Sadr & Capps, 1992; Fauci, 1989; Zahner, Oliver, & Siemering, 2014). Additionally, Sengupta and colleagues (2000) performed a study aimed at understanding the factors affecting participation in AIDS-related research by African Americans and found that distrust in scientists and research institutions was a major factor contributing to individuals' unwillingness to participate (Shavers-Hornaday et al., 1997). Other researchers have found this mistrust of researchers among African Americans—especially those in the rural South—appears to be rooted in the historical events of the Tuskegee Syphilis Study (Berkley-Patton, 2013; Freimuth et al., 2001; George, Duran, & Norris, 2014; Sengupta et al., 2000) This phenomenon has been confirmed by anecdotal evidence from our interactions with PLWHA in the rural South.

Therefore, community engagement—defined by the Centers for Disease Control and Prevention (2011) as "the process of working collaboratively with groups of people who are affiliated by geographic proximity, special interests, or similar situations with respect to issues affecting their well-being"—was the cornerstone of all the research activities we engaged in. Given our experience (Scharff et al., 2010), from the beginning we set out to create a broad and inclusive team involving interdisciplinary researchers, community leaders, peer leaders, and research staff. Importantly, in forming our collaboration, we prioritized the acknowledgment of each team member's unique knowledge and expertise. Equally important was the need to foster an atmosphere of shared responsibility, where each individual's expertise and strengths are equitably utilized to achieve the overall goal of the project. Currently, the core members of our team include interdisciplinary researchers at the University of Alabama (George Mugoya, PhD, MPH, an associate professor of rehabilitation counseling; Safiya George, PhD, an associate professor and assistant dean for research at Capstone College of Nursing; and Pamela Payne-Foster, MD, MPH, a professor of medicine), a community leader in charge of a nongovernmental organization offering services for PLWHA in West Alabama (Billy Kirkpatrick, PhD, chief executive officer, Five Horizons Health System), and peer leaders.

As we said above, an important aspect of our collaboration was understanding the unique characteristics of each team member. In the initial phases of forming our partnership, the interdisciplinary researchers and community leader attended training on grant funding led by

David G. Bauer. During the training, Bauer had team members participate in Allen N. Fahden and Srinivasan Namakkal's Innovate with C.A.R.E. Profile (Bauer, 2011). This profile is completed individually by team members and clarifies the role(s) that each member prefers during team processes. A description is then provided for how each role preference shapes an individual team member's thought and behavior patterns. The profiles gave team members insight into the thoughts and subsequent behaviors of other members and also suggested roles that would be most comfortable for each team member. For instance, Safiya George was identified as a *Refiner* who generates ideas, improves ideas before implementation, and plans implementation. Billy Kirkpatrick was identified as an *Advancer/Executor* who promotes team objectives, defines tasks and methods, ensures that solutions are implemented in an orderly manner, and advances new directions. George Mugoya, as a *Refiner/Executor*, determines that concepts and details are thoroughly assessed prior to implementation, ensures that plans are carried out in an orderly manner, improves on ideas, and develops detailed implementation plans. Pamela Payne-Foster was identified as a *Creator/Refiner* and, as such, generates concepts and ideas, perceives the "big picture," and challenges concepts under discussion to make sure that concepts are examined thoroughly. The knowledge gained from this assessment allowed team members to merge previously known strengths with newly identified thought and behavior patterns. The benefits of integrating such knowledge related to oneself and others have been, and continue to be, carried into our various research endeavors.

Relevant Projects

As a team we have been engaged in various research projects aimed at improving the quality of life for our target population. We concentrate on multilevel strategies to improve HIV/AIDS outcomes and a related project to improve mental health outcomes for PLWHA by using telehealth. The goal of multilevel-strategies to improve HIV/AIDS outcomes was to ascertain how to better offer group counseling services for PLWHA with comorbid substance use and mental health issues. A majority of our clients were in rural areas; thus, transportation was an issue. Relatedly, participants from the rural areas had indicated reservations about attending counseling where they might be recognized and thus risked their HIV diagnosis being known. We considered telehealth as a means to conduct counseling as it would address both transportation issues and the concern for anonymity of our clients. During this project, we learned important lessons about offering counseling utilizing telehealth including addressing issues related to internet connectivity in the rural areas. Results indicated that counseling via telehealth was as effective as counseling face to face if certain conditions supported client confidence. For example, the team noted that the patients need to establish a relationship with the counselor, which may require offering at least one face-to-face counseling session. The successes and lessons learned from this project have been utilized by our partner agency—Five Horizons Health Services—in implementing individual counseling for PLWHA with self-reported mental health and/or substance abuse issues. We plan to expand the project and offer case management services via telehealth.

Recruiting Peer Leaders

As noted, our research projects include full participation by PLWHA in order that the process be authentically community-engaged and informed by those we are attempting to serve through the research. It is also important that team members be keenly aware of the mistrust felt by traditionally stigmatized populations toward researchers (George, Duran, & Norris, 2014). Based on these factors, the decision was made to include peer leadership—specifically, those who live with HIV—as an integral and equal component of the research team.

To assist with the formation of the peer leadership team, Payne-Foster facilitated a previously developed framework for training. The training program included both a full-day training seminar and continuous mentorship by both research and community leaders. Given the pilot nature of the project, we relied on our community partner, Five Horizons Health Services, to recommend potential peer leaders. Among the attributes we sought for potential peer leaders were: (a) being HIV positive, (b) being consistent with HIV/AIDS treatment, and (c) having demonstrated potential for leadership and advocacy skills within the HIV community (e.g., active participation in the Alabama HIV Advocacy Day events). The one-day peer leadership training provided an in-depth description of peer leadership, discussed social issues related to HIV/AIDS, and allowed for the practice of facilitation skills. A group of four individuals meeting the eligibility criteria were identified by our partner agency and recruited. All four attended the training seminar, and two have consistently participated in our research projects. Unfortunately, one of our trained peer leaders developed serious disease and had to step aside. This brings to fore that despite the fact that effective antiretroviral therapy is slowing progression to AIDS, some individuals with HIV are still facing serious health problems.

Notwithstanding, our active peer leaders remained dynamic and connected with the community. The peers have spent years meeting the social needs of PLWHA, including the provision of transportation. They also lead statewide advocacy efforts, acting as mentors for PLWHA who are unfamiliar with the process. They are also skilled at connecting researchers to staff at various AIDS service organizations.

The Power of Peer Leadership

The inclusion of peer leaders paid immediate dividends, as they have a longstanding history of trust and good rapport with both the HIV community and HIV providers in the region. A prominent example of the impact of peer leaders is evident in a current project, Project CHAP (Case Management, Housing, Advocacy, and Policy). This project, which requires lengthy interviews and the discussion of deeply personal information from PLWHA, is heavily aided by the presence of peer leaders. Participants have no prior relationship with researchers and often deny requests for participation when solicited solely by researchers. However, peer leaders, based on the strength of personal relationships, are able to bridge the gap between participants and researchers, thereby increasing participation in research and the comfort that participants feel during the process. Peer leaders were equal partners in our projects and were included in all aspects of the project including the development of the interview protocols. Indeed, peers provided alternate perspectives for researchers to consider regarding recruitment, study procedures, and covariates. Involving peer leaders in all aspects of the study has provided meaningful insight into the day-to-day issues faced by PLWHA in the rural South that might serve as barriers to care and barriers to HIV-related research and policy activities. Their participation also highlights the importance of examining multiple perspectives when addressing these issues.

Research Staff

In addition to peer leaders, employing qualified and motivated project staff has been integral as research team members do not generally have the time necessary to manage all the details of project facilitation. The most important staff role has been that of project coordinator, who is responsible for the completion of all relevant consents and surveys, the provision of regular status reports, and the maintenance of open communication between principal investigators (PIs), community partners, peer leaders, research assistants (RAs), participants, and recruitment sites. In the previous three years, the role of project coordinator has been held by four individuals. (While this may appear to be a high turnover, it is noteworthy that two of the project coordinators were recruited from the RAs to ensure the continuity and maintenance of the relationships we had established. The RAs who took this position were in the final year of their program and left the program after graduation.) The program coordinators, along with numerous research assistants, have brought unique perspectives and skills to the research process, and each has been able to develop a uniquely personal rapport with study participants.

Lessons Learned, Conclusions, and Implications

For individuals in the rural South, being diagnosed with a stigmatizing condition such as HIV/AIDS can have immense implications in their lives, including a decision to leave the homes they have known all their lives. The ongoing collaborations described here highlight the necessity of having wide and inclusive collaborations that involve researchers, community members, and PLWHA. A very important aspect of current research projects has been the inclusion of peer leaders in the process of designing and implementing the project, which has facilitated optimal engagement by participants who are PLWHA across the state. It is also important to facilitate the development of peer leaders by offering tailored training. Training for peer leaders is essential to rebuild communication and trust between academic researchers and the HIV community. The role of peer leaders in community-based research is unique in that they often share lived experiences with and exert influence on participants' decisions. In addition, as peer leaders who help others navigate HIV resources, they are able to identify barriers to PLWHA seeking care, staying in care, and obtaining optimal viral suppression.

One of the most important lessons learned from our work is that to form truly collaborative relationships, team members need to understand each other's strengths and weaknesses and work collaboratively to harness every team member's strengths. Additionally, recruiting a project coordinator proved to be essential in ensuring all resources were managed efficiently and all project scheduling and activities were appropriately coordinated. Scheduling and facilitating team meetings has been a critical part of the process, allowing us the opportunity to provide project updates, discuss challenges, and identify solutions and next steps. Lastly, it's vital to actively involve participants, especially peer leaders, in all aspects of the research project.

A case could be made that these collaborations will become the standard for community-based research. Substantive collaborations among all HIV/AIDS stakeholders in the rural South can have important implications for both treatment and policies such as bringing about changes in the formula for Housing Opportunities for Persons with AIDS (HOPWA) funding. Such collaborations among stakeholders need to be fostered.

We are hopeful that our collaborative research efforts will lay the groundwork for future research and policy work in the area of housing and case management among PLWHA in the rural South. This is important work (see George Dalmida et al., 2019), which focuses on forming substantive collaborations that involve all stakeholders with the goal of reducing health disparities in the rural South and improving health outcomes of individuals with HIV/AIDS, one of the most stigmatized groups of individuals in the United States. Further, as indicated above, our work has afforded us an opportunity to assess the potential and challenges associated with providing telehealth counseling. While Five Horizons Health Services is at the early phases of implementing telehealth to provide services, we believe that the long-term effects of this research could have great significance.

References

Adimora, A. A., Schoenbach, V. J., Martinson, F. E., Donaldson, K. H., Stancil, T. R., & Fullilove, R. E. (2003). Concurrent partnerships among rural African Americans with recently reported heterosexually transmitted HIV infection. *Journal of Acquired Immune Deficiency Syndrome, 34*(4), 423–429.

Alabama Department of Public Health (ADPH). (2019). *Brief facts on African Americans and HIV in Alabama*. Retrieved August 2, 2021, from https://www.alabamapublichealth.gov/hiv/assets/brieffactsonafricanamericansandhiv.pdf

Bauer, D. G. (2011). *The "how to" grants manual: Successful grantseeking techniques for obtaining public and private grants* (7th ed.). Rowman & Littlefield.

Berkley-Patton, J. Y., Moore, E., Berman, M., Simon, S. D., Thompson, C. B, Schleicher, T., & Hawes, S. M. (2013). Assessment of HIV-related stigma in a U.S. faith-based HIV education and testing intervention. *Journal of the International AIDS Society, 16*(2), 18644. https://doi.org/10.7448/IAS.16.3.18644

Centers for Disease Control and Prevention (CDC). (2011). *Principles of community engagement* (2nd ed.). Retrieved February 3, 2013, from https://www.atsdr.cdc.gov/community engagement/pdf/PCE_Report_508_FINAL.pdf

Centers for Disease Control and Prevention (CDC). (2012). *HIV in the United States: The stages of care.* Retrieved February 3, 2013, from https://www.cdc.gov/hiv/pdf/research_mmp_stagesofcare.pdf

Centers for Disease Control and Prevention (CDC). (2014). *National Center for HIV/AIDS, Viral Hepatitis C, STD, and TB Prevention (NCHHSTP) atlas.* Retrieved July 2016, from http://www.cdc.gov/nchhstp/atlas/

Earnshaw, V. A., Bogart, L. M., Dovidio, J. F., & Williams, D. R. (2013). Stigma and racial/ethnic HIV disparities: Moving toward resilience. *American Psychologist, 68*(4), 225–236. https://doi.org/10.1037/a0032705

El-Sadr, W., & Capps, L. (1992). The challenge of minority recruitment in clinical trials for AIDS. *Journal of American Medical Association, 267*(7), 954–957.

Emlet, C. A. (2005). Measuring stigma in older and younger adults with HIV/AIDS: An analysis of an HIV stigma scale and initial exploration of subscales. *Research on Social Work Practice, 15*(4), 291–300.

Fauci, A. S. (1989). AIDS—challenges to basic and clinical biomedical research. *Academic Medicine, 64*(3), 115–119.

Foster, P. H. (2007). Use of stigma, fear, and denial in development of a framework for prevention of HIV/AIDS in rural African American communities. *Family and Community Health, 30*(4), 318–327.

Foster, P. P., & Gaskins, S. W. (2009). Older African Americans' management of HIV/AIDS stigma. *AIDS Care, 21*(10), 1306–1312.

Foster, P. P., Thomas, M., & Lewis, D. (2016). Reverse migration, the Black church, and sexual health: Implications for building HIV/AIDS prevention capacity in the Deep South. *AIMS Public Health, 3*(2), 242–254.

Freimuth, V. S., Quinn, S. C., Thomas, S. B., Cole, G., Zook, E., & Duncan, T. (2001). African Americans' views on research and the Tuskegee Syphilis Study. *Social Science & Medicine, 52*(5), 797–808.

George, S., Duran, N., & Norris, K. (2014). A systematic review of barriers and facilitators to minority research participation among African Americans, Latinos, Asian Americans, and Pacific Islanders. *American Journal of Public Health, 104*(2), e16–e31.

George Dalmida, S., Mugoya, G. C., Kirkpatrick, B., Kraemer, K. R., Bonner, F., Merritt, J., & Muiga, W. (2019). Interdisciplinary, community, and peer leadership approach to addressing housing among people living with HIV in the rural South. *Housing Policy Debate, 29*(3), 462–474.

Hawes-Dawson, J., Derose, K. P., Aunon, F. M, Dominguez, B. X., Felton, A., Mata, M. A., Oden, C. W., & Paffen, S. (2017). Achieving broad participation in congregant health surveys in African American and Latino churches. *Field Methods, 29*(1), 79–94.

Herek, G. (1999). AIDS and stigma. *AIDS and Behavior, 42*(7), 1106–1116.

Herek, G. M., Capitanio, J. P., & Widaman, K. F. (2002). HIV-related stigma and knowledge in the United States: Prevalence and trends, 1991–1999. *American Journal of Public Health, 92*(3), 371–377. https://doi.org/10.2105/AJPH.92.3.371

Horstmann, E., Brown, J., Islam, F., Buck, J., & Again, B. D. (2010). Retaining HIV-infected patients in care: Where are we? Where do we go from here? *Clinical Infectious Diseases, 50*(5), 752–761.

Lichtenstein, B. (2007). Illicit drug use and the social context of HIV/AIDS in Alabama's Black Belt. *Journal of Rural Health, 23*(1), 68–72.

Lindley, L. L., Coleman, J. D., & Gaddist, B. W. (2010). Informing faith-based HIV/AIDS interventions: HIV-related knowledge and stigmatizing attitudes at Project F.A.I.T.H. churches in South Carolina. *Public Health Reports, 125*(1), 12–20.

Magnus, M., Jones, K., Phillips, G., Binson, D., Hightow-Weidman, L. B., Richards-Clarke, C., Wohl, A. R., Outlaw, A., Giordano, T. P., Quamina, A., Cobbs, W., Fields, S. D., Tinsley, M., Cajina, A., & Hidalgo, J. (2010). Characteristics associated with retention among African American and Latino adolescent HIV positive men: Results from the outreach, care, and prevention to engage HIV-seropositive young MSM of color special project of national significance initiative. *Journal of Acquired Immune Deficiency Syndrome, 53*, 529–536.

Mahajan, A., Sayles, J., Patel, V., Remien, R. H., Sawires, S. R., Ortiz, D. J., Szekeres, G., & Coates, T. J. (2008). Stigma in the HIV/AIDS epidemic: A review of the literature and recommendations for the way forward. *AIDS, 22*(2), S67–S79.

Mugavero, M. J., Amico, K. R., Horn, T., Thompson, M. A. (2013). The state of engagement in HIV care in the United States: From cascade to continuum to control. *Clinical Infectious Disease, 57*(8), 1164–1171.

Nelson, A. (2002). Unequal treatment: Confronting racial and ethnic disparities in health care. *Journal of the National Medical Association, 94*(8), 666–668.

Nunn, A., Cornwall, A., Thomas, G., Calahan, P. L, Waller, P. A., Friend, R., Broadnax, P. J., & Flanigan, T. (2013). What's God got to do with it? Engaging

African-American faith-based institutions in HIV prevention. *Global Public Health, 8*(3), 258–269.

Payne-Foster, P., Bradley, E.L.P., Aduloju-Ajijola N., Yang, X., Gaul, Z., Parton, J., Sutton, M. Y., & Gaskins, S. (2018). Testing our FAITH: HIV stigma and knowledge after a faith-based HIV stigma reduction intervention in the rural South. *AIDS Care, 30*(2), 232–239.

Plumb, J., Weinstein, L. C., Brawer, R., & Scott, K. (2012). Community-based partnerships for improving chronic disease management. *Primary Care, 39*(2), 433–447.

Reif, S., Safley, D., McAllaster, C., Wilson, E., & Whetten, K. (2017). State of HIV in the US Deep South. *Journal of Community Health, 42*(5), 844–853.

Reif, S., Safley, D., Wilson, E., & Whetten, K. (2016, January). HIV/AIDS in the U.S. Deep South: Trends from 2008–2013. Retrieved February 3, 2016, from https://southernaids.files.wordpress.com/2011/10/hiv-aids-in-the-us-deep-south-trends-from-2008–2013.pdf

Scharff, D. P., Matthews, K. P., Jackson, P., Hoffsuemmer, J., Martin, E., & Edwards, D. (2010). More than Tuskegee: Understanding mistrust about research participation. *Journal of Health Care for the Poor and Underserved, 21*(3), 879–897.

Sengupta, S., Strauss, R. P., DeVellis, R., Quinn, S. C., DeVellis, B., & Ware, W. B. (2000). Factors affecting African-American participation in AIDS research. *Journal of Acquired Immune Deficiency Syndrome, 24*(3), 275–284.

Shavers-Hornaday, V. L., Lynch, C. F., Burmeister, L. F., & Torner, J. C. (1997). Why are African Americans under-represented in medical research studies? Impediments to participation. *Ethnicity & Health, 2*(1/2), 31–45.

Smith, J., Simmons, E., & Mayer, K. H. (2005). HIV/AIDS and the Black church: What are the barriers to prevention services? *Journal of the National Medical Association, 97*(12), 1682–1685.

Warf, B., & Winsberg, M. (2008). The geography of religious diversity in the United States. *Professional Geographer, 60*(3), 413–424.

Williams, D. R., & Mohammed, S. A. (2009). Discrimination and racial disparities in health: Evidence and needed research. *Journal of Behavioral Medicine, 32*(1), 20–47.

Zahner, S. J., Oliver, T. R., & Siemering, K. Q. (2014, January 9). The mobilizing action toward community health partnership study: Multisector partnerships in U.S. counties with improving health metrics. *Preventing Chronic Disease: Public Health Research, Practice, and Policy, 11*. http://dx.doi.org/10.5888/pcd11.130103

Chapter 3

Making Baton Rouge Better

No Longer a Tale of Two Cities

Leslie T. Grover and Revathi I. Hines

The authors of this chapter are both members of the Baton Rouge, Louisiana, community. We are also members of marginalized communities there. Our work and our lived experiences have shown us how important it is to try to bridge the racial divide in Baton Rouge. Leslie T. Grover's background in public policy, narrative medicine, and community-based participatory research has given her the desire to make community voices drivers of community policy. It has also motivated her to seek out those voices that are mostly unheard. Revathi I. Hines's background in political science and in narrative therapy, too, helps the team focus on stories, healing, and vulnerable communities. Her desire to make an impact drives her to make positive changes in vulnerable communities.

Using Community Conversations and a Restorative Justice model support our objectives. Meetings, encounters, discussions, and sharing narratives create empathy and break down walls. They lead to understanding and shared senses of community.

In doing this work, we learned that there are differences in how policy-makers and community members view health, housing, and race. But we also learned that the unheard voices need opportunities to contribute. We think things went well, but we want to see more marginalized voices at the table. To achieve this end, we have learned that we must take the work to the people we want involved. We must continue to build trust in the margins of the community by participating and respecting mores, working with community partners, and being a constant presence. It is not the responsibility of those who have been disenfranchised or left out to seek out our opportunities. Rather it is our responsibility to seek them out and to work with them on their own terms and in their own spaces. As you read this chapter, note the importance of the community voice as a driver of the work.

Race, space, and place have been both a curse and a blessing in Baton Rouge, Louisiana. As a blessing, these elements make it easy for people to speak candidly to one another, even in times of distress. As a curse, these same elements have often calcified generations of mistrust and inequality, and in so doing have systematically excluded many community members from important decisions in the city. In this chapter, we discuss our attempts to use the power of conversation and sharing personal stories in making Baton Rouge a city more united and communal in addressing its racial and health disparities. Our Community Conversations are the focus here, and we spent months in the community conducting this powerful series.

Baton Rouge is a city that is a prototype for both the foundations of unrest and a cautionary tale about the socioeconomic consequences of racism. The interplay of community systems such as education, health, employment, and involvement in the justice system have critical implications for community well-being. As Schultz and Northridge (2004) point out, how health, education, employment, and law enforcement complexly interplay can determine the risk of communities of becoming more at risk: the physical environment is shaped by the social interactions of community members; those patterns are strongly influenced by economics and by values linked to race and ethnicity; these interactions affect health outcomes; and the interconnections of those connections influence the overall survival of the community. However, there is also another level of interactions that shape community outcomes in Baton Rouge, and that is policy decisions. Though race is a social construct, the combined effect of social interactions and policy decisions is a powerful one when it comes to how community members identify.

Like most communities in the Deep South, Baton Rouge has a history of the enslavement and mistreatment of Black people and housing patterns that are driven by racism, segregation, and discrimination. The city is among the most racially segregated in the nation (Louisiana Network, 2017). Deslatte (2016) describes the division in the city: "In Baton Rouge, an invisible, informal line segregates the community, dividing the southern White section from the mostly black part in the north. Breakaway school districts have formed. Some in the south end want to take things further by breaking off completely and forming a new city."

North Baton Rouge lacks commercial development. The benefits of previous economic wins—a once thriving film industry, hotel construction, and major investments by such technology firms as IBM and EA Games—have mostly accrued in the southern part of the city. And efforts by one or two local politicians to improve the northern part of the city have been met with great protest by their policymaking peers. As Brown (2016) points out, to the extent that lawmakers have tried to spark progress in that area, it has largely had no measurable gains to report. The one main attraction in the northern part of the city is the Baton Rouge Zoo.

The zoo has lost accreditation and suffers from neglect, and the principal proposal from zoo leadership to improve it was moving the zoo from northern Baton Rouge to the southern part of the city. With the help of mayors and residents from surrounding smaller communities (Baker, Zachary, and Central) and the leadership of one councilwoman whose district would have been hardest hit by the zoo's relocation, the public backlash grew enough to lead the managing board of the zoo to reject the proposal to move the facility (Gallo, 2018).

Educational outcomes for Black people in the city lag behind their White counterparts. Fewer than one in ten residents in the city describe the educational options in the city as "excellent," and as charter schools proliferate in the city, public schools lose funding as students seek better education opportunities elsewhere (Baton Rouge Area Foundation, 2016). Economic opportunity for Black community members lag as well. Black people in the area are three times more likely to experience poverty than their White counterparts (Citydata.com, 2016). Black people are less likely to be hired than White people in the city, even if they are equally or overly qualified. Black families have been separated as well-educated children have had to move to other cities in search of jobs (Deslatte, 2016).

These economic disparities have greatly contributed to health disparities. There is a twelve-year difference between the lifespans of Black people who live in the northern part of the city and their White counterparts in the southern part of the city. Access to healthcare, including behavioral health resources, bears out a disheartening story along racial lines. Over the past decade the state dismantled the charity health system that had provided affordable healthcare to thousands, particularly in underserved areas. In 2013, Baton Rouge witnessed the closing of Earl K. Long Medical Center, a charity-system medical facility located in North Baton Rouge, one of the poorest parts of the city. Not only did the hospital serve poor, uninsured, and underinsured residents, it also served as home to a mental health emergency room, a twenty-bed facility that served as a temporary stop for people in need of mental health treatment. Patients were stabilized at the hospital and then referred or transferred to mental health clinics, hospitals, or other services. Baton Rouge reflects mental health access across the state of Louisiana, which consistently has ranked in the bottom when it comes to mental health outcomes and access to services. Louisiana currently ranks forty-fifth of the fifty states (Mental Health America, 2018).

The justice system also reflects race-based disparities. The state of Louisiana has the highest incarceration rate in the nation, with the vast majority of inmates identifying as Black. Trends in Baton Rouge reflect this, with Black people getting incarcerated at nearly three times the rate of White people for similar crimes. Further, the Vera Institute of Justice (2015) reports that approximately three of every four inmates in East Baton Rouge Parish jail are Black. Though the city is nearly 60 percent Black, the police force does not reflect those demographics or connections to the local community. Two of every three police officers in the city are White, and the department has struggled for decades to diversify the force (Fausset et al., 2016). In fact, the city is still under a consent decree which is over thirty years old that mandates creating opportunities for more Black officers to join the force. It remains one of the most racially disparate forces in the nation (Berube & Holmes, 2016).

Hell Summer

The divisions between Black and White people in the city intensified during the summer of 2016, often referred to locally as "Hell Summer," with the interplay of three major events: the murder of Alton Sterling by police, the ambush of law enforcement officers by a lone gunman, and the Great Flood. These events happened within weeks of each other, and they have altered the city's race relations. Traumatic events cut more deeply because of the narratives that grow up around them, narratives that solidify divisions and rub salt into racial wounds. Race relations have polarized Baton Rouge even more in the wake of Hell Summer, not just with implications for those who have been discriminated against, like the Black population of the city, but also for the White members of the community, both those who have actively participated in racism and those who have not.

On July 5, 2016, Alton Sterling, a thirty-seven-year-old Black man, was selling CDs outside of a local convenience store when he was approached by a homeless man who asked him for money. Sterling refused, but the homeless man persisted. After refusing several more pleas for money, Sterling brandished a gun, admonishing the man to leave him alone. The man left the scene and called 9–1–1, reporting that Sterling had threatened him with a gun. Several minutes later two White police officers, Blane Salamoni and Howie Lake II, arrived on the scene. Salamoni yelled expletives at Sterling upon arrival, and the officers wrestled him to the ground. Six minutes later, a cell phone camera captured the struggle, including Sterling being tased and eventually shot by Salamoni, who fired six times. Three of the shots were in Sterling's back. The city ignited as mostly Black local residents protested, demanding justice for the police killing of Sterling. Sterling's family and the local NAACP held a press conference, calling for the resignation of Carl Dabadie, the White police chief. Dabadie refused to resign.

The two police officers were immediately placed on paid leave, and a day later, Governor John Bel Edwards turned over the case to the FBI and the Department of Justice. The district attorney, Hilar Moore, recused himself from the case, citing a close personal relationship with the Salamoni family. Protests continued, mostly in the northern parts of the city, with the city arresting thousands of Black protesters.

Nearly ten days later and on his birthday—July 17, 2016—a military veteran from Dallas, Texas, named Gavin Long entered Baton Rouge near a small strip mall. Armed with several guns, Long shot four law enforcement officers. The shooting left three officers dead: East Baton Rouge sheriff's deputy Brad Garafola and Baton Rouge police officers Montrell Jackson and Matthew Gerald. A fourth police officer, Deputy Nicholas Tullier, was badly injured. Long was killed by police, and many in Baton Rouge surmised the attack on officers was retaliation, even though Long's suicide note did not mention Sterling specifically. He did allude to problems between police officers and Black people. The letter said his actions were a "necessary evil" that he hoped would compel good officers to work to reform the system to get rid of bad officers who were attacking and killing "his people" (Brown, 2016). Though one of the murdered law enforcement officers, Montrell Jackson, was Black, the city again picked sides in the police shootings. In the southern part of the city, White businesses and residents placed Blue Lives Matter bumper stickers and flags on their homes and cars. As was the case in many cities, this was a direct response to the Black Lives Matter chants at protests for Alton Sterling, socially signaling White aversion to Black community members challenging the status quo of racial inequality (Cooper, 2020).

Almost a month later, while the city was still deeply divided over the killings of both Sterling and the three law enforcement officers, the weather began to change. On August 9, 2016, the small community north of Baton Rouge proper began to flood. A few families left their homes, and by the end of the week on August 12, another northern section of the area flooded, leaving thousands of residents without homes and businesses. The city scrambled to evacuate residents and to help those who had flooded move to higher ground. By August 15, all but the southern-most part of the city flooded. Residents and experts alike were caught unprepared as flooding of such magnitude was described as so unlikely that it would happen only once every thousand years. But it happened in Baton Rouge during Hell Summer. The Great Flood of 2016 inundated the greater Baton Rouge area with over 7 trillion gallons of rain falling in the area in just thirty-six hours, causing an estimated $20.7 billion in property damage. Approximately 31 percent of homes, or more than 100,000 homes, in the region were damaged or destroyed; only 11 percent of households had flood insurance. Approximately 6,000 businesses flooded and more than 278,000 workers were not able to go to work. The August storm claimed thirteen lives (Gallo & Russell, 2016). Many are still in the process of rebuilding after the flood in 2016, and many homes and small businesses have been abandoned and sold altogether.

In the aftermath of the Alton Sterling shooting, the police shootings, and the Great Flood, the city has undergone drastic changes. The unincorporated, financially thriving, southernmost part of East Baton Rouge Parish attempted to found a new city—St. George—alongside the city of Baton Rouge. Currently, many Baton Rouge residents don't actually live in the city proper—they live in "unincorporated areas" within the parish, basically indistinguishable from the sprawling city (Brown, 2016). Louisiana law allows these areas to organize as cities of their own, provided enough people sign a petition to get on the ballot. It is this law that has allowed other smaller communities in the area to form their own community school systems.

However, unlike other efforts that have resulted in smaller, Whiter off-shoots from Baton Rouge proper, the St. George effort is more contrived. Black households have been deliberately cut out, often dividing neighborhoods in strange ways that would divide residents who live just inches from each other into two different jurisdictions. Further, the boundaries would attempt to take the major economic engines in that part of the city, such as a large shopping mall and the two largest and most advanced hospitals, right along with it. While proponents vehemently deny that race is a factor, it is hard to ignore the fact that Black households have been carved out of the area almost completely (Harris, 2019).

After several attempts, this measure has finally passed. If projections are correct, 30 percent of the parish general fund will vanish, since wealthier citizens now live in the new city. Further, this city will all but destroy the financial well-being of the city of Baton Rouge and north Baton Rouge in particular. Racially the city will flip the demographics of Baton Rouge. St. George will be 70 percent White, 23 percent Black (Brown, 2016).

Baton Rouge's Historical Trauma

In Baton Rouge racism plays a major role in influencing housing availability, educational outcomes, and job opportunities. However, there is another aspect to the polarizing effects of racism important to understanding the backdrop of our work in Baton Rouge—historical trauma.

Trauma is derived from the Greek term for "wound." Exceedingly frightening or distressing events may result in a psychological wound or injury, which can translate into difficulty in coping or functioning normally following a particular event or experience. The same event or experience may have little impact on one person but may cause severe distress in another. The impact that an event has may be related to the person's mental and physical health, level of available support at the time of the event, and past experience and coping skills, or to a person's sense of self. Complex trauma happens when adversity is experienced over a prolonged period of time, or when different adversities are repeated within a given period of time, or when adversities have a cumulative effect on an individual's life course. These adversities can include conditions such as poverty and ongoing economic concerns about a lack of basic essentials such as food, water, shelter, and safety; community violence and economic isolation; homelessness; incarceration; poor-quality housing; or political, social, and economic disenfranchisement based on race, ethnicity, religious practices, etc. (Bartlett et al., 2018).

When complex trauma is experienced over the course of generations it is known as historical trauma. Historical trauma refers to a complex and collective trauma experienced over time and across generations by a group of people who share an identity, affiliation, or circumstance (Mohatt et al., 2014). Historical trauma can be understood as consisting of three primary elements. First is the trauma itself. Second is that the trauma is shared by a group of people, rather than being individually experienced. Third, the trauma spans multiple generations, even though subsequent members of the affected group were not present for the past traumatizing event (Mohatt et al., 2014). Krieger (2001) recognizes three theories that underpin current understanding of historical trauma. The first is psychosocial theory, which deliberately links physical and psychological stress with the social environment. The second theoretical framework is political/economic theory, which addresses the political, economic, and structural determinants such as unjust power relations and class inequality. The third is social/ecological systems theory, which recognizes the multilevel dynamics and interdependencies of present/past, proximate/distal, and life-course factors.

Historical trauma theory, then, provides a macro-level framework for understanding how the "life course" of a population exposed to trauma at a particular point in time compares with that of unexposed populations.

Danieli (1998) breaks down the components of complex and historical trauma into three distinct categories: the historical trauma experience, the historical trauma response, and the intergenerational transmission of historical trauma. Historical trauma has expensive social consequences. In 2013, for example, the W. K. Kellogg Foundation conducted a study focused on the intersection of race, class, residential segregation, and income disparity. The study found the income gap created by racism costs the United States nearly $2 trillion per year. Further, if racial income inequality alone was eliminated, the study finds, the purchasing power of minorities would increase from $4.3 trillion to $6.1 trillion by 2045. In 2016 Pettus-Davis et al. (2018) studied the social costs of mass incarceration and its disproportionate effects on Black families in the United States. They found that for every dollar mass incarceration costs, it creates $10 in social costs. These social costs are borne most by Black women and in Black neighborhoods across the nation (Roberts, 2003). This is certainly true in Baton Rouge, where Black members of the community are the most likely to pay the highest social costs.

Yehuda et al. (2007, 2008, 2009, 2014, 2016) have studied historical trauma and how it can be transmitted intergenerationally from a biological standpoint. She and her colleagues examined how historical traumas such as slavery and the Holocaust and the subsequent stress can be passed down through generations in shared family genes. Her research has revealed that when people experience trauma, it changes their genes in a very specific and noticeable way so that when those people have children and their genes are passed down to their children, the children also inherit the genes affected by trauma. The genes are carried from the maternal side of the family and can have devastating social effects. Theories of historical trauma recognize that populations traditionally subjected to long-term, mass trauma—colonialism, slavery, war, genocide—exhibit a higher prevalence of disease and other negative health factors for at least several generations after the original trauma occurred (Sotero, 2006). These prevalences carry with them high social costs, private costs, and community costs.

Sotero (2006) recognizes four distinct assumptions regarding historical trauma: (1) mass trauma is deliberately and systematically inflicted upon a target population by a subjugating, dominant population; (2) trauma is not limited to a single catastrophic event, but continues over an extended period of time (complex trauma); (3) traumatic events reverberate throughout the population, creating a universal experience of trauma; and (4) the magnitude of the trauma experience derails the population from its natural, projected historical course resulting in a legacy of physical, psychological, social, and economic disparities that persists across generations.

As Mohatt and colleagues (2014) explain: "Historical trauma functions as a public narrative for particular groups or communities that connects present-day experiences and circumstances to the trauma. Treating historical trauma as a public narrative shifts the research discourse away from an exclusive search for past causal variables to identifying how present-day experiences, their corresponding narratives, and their health impacts are connected to public narratives of historical trauma for a particular group or community" (p. 128).

Addressing Historical Trauma at the Community Level through Storytelling

While much of the literature on emotional trauma focuses on the individual, a growing number of practitioners and academics have also recognized trauma can be experienced at the community level. So far, however, there is not a common framework that allows practitioners, community leaders, or residents to address the effects of complex traumas like those experienced in Baton Rouge such as racism, violence, poverty, and segregation (Pinderhughes, Davis, & Williams, 2015).

What we know from our work is that addressing historical trauma at the community level is much more nuanced than at the individual level. Communities are more unpredictable. They have the interplay of several interrelated components that make its trauma particularly complex: the people; the place; the informal interactions among people in the place, including infrastructure and public services; and the opportunities to interact that come about in the local economy and other institutions.

A useful approach for Baton Rouge and similar communities at least recognizes the effects of racism and the institutional consequences of it. These can manifest in a number of ways and in a number of community institutions. As Pinderhughes, Davis, and Williams (2015) point out, "Community trauma is not just the aggregate of individuals in a neighborhood who have experienced trauma from exposures to violence. There are manifestations, or symptoms, of community trauma at the community level. The symptoms are present in the social-cultural environment, the physical/built environment and the economic environment." Further, "communities, like the members and families that inhabit them, are dynamic rather than static. As living systems, they face opportunities, as well as challenges—some expected and some unexpected. At any one point in time, communities face a unique combination of situations and events, demands and hardships, and resources and opportunities in the context of contemporary circumstances, historical events and actions, and an unfolding future" (Mancini & Bowen, 2009).

The Community Conversation Series

We believe that the Restorative Justice Institute's encounter approach would greatly benefit Baton Rouge as the community seeks ways to more effectively address the effects of racism that are woven into its fabric. A restorative encounter has five interwoven elements, three of which are discussed here (Van Ness & Strong, 2003). Each of these elements contributes to the strength of the encounter. Meeting is about engagement of all parties involved. Narrative involves community members describing what happened to them regarding racism, how that has affected them, and how they view racism and its consequences. Lastly is agreement. Encounter programs seek a resolution that fits the immediate parties rather than focusing on a permanent or one-size-fits-all solution.

Because communities are dynamic, the encounter approach opens up the possibility of designing a uniquely crafted resolution reflecting the circumstances of the Baton Rouge community. Further, the approach does this through a cooperative process rather than an adversarial one, through negotiation that searches for a convergence of the interests of residents from both the northern and southern parts of the city, and through the ability to guide the outcome.

In less polarized communities the elements of people, place, informal interactions and formal interactions in the market can promote and sustain community health and safety and foster a sense of belonging and ownership among community members. When a community is as traumatized like Baton Rouge is, however, each of the elements as well as the interplay of those elements is damaged. This damage begins to perpetuate the problems rather than community well-being. In these circumstances these factors can contribute to inequities in health, housing, education, and other determinants of the well-being of community members instead of healing them. This was the case in Baton Rouge before Hell Summer. The deepening racial polarization in Baton Rouge is a product of decades of economic, political, and social disenfranchisement, a lack of investment in the economic development of the northern part of the city, and the loss of social capital with the flight of many middle-class families to outlying areas.

The propensity for Black residents to experience the negative outcomes of the disparities that exist in the Baton Rouge community over and over underscores a particular need for a recognition that such experiences have contributed to, for example, the increased likelihood of becoming involved in the justice system. A healthy community intervention understands social inequality as a structural condition, and not a personal characteristic, and it does this alongside awareness of and sensitivity to the dynamics of historical trauma, in all aspects of the planning, formulation, and evaluation of policies and programming meant to address some of the social and economic consequences of historical trauma on community members.

One of the most effective ways to solicit perspectives with encounters is through the use of narratives. Narratives serve as the basis for sharing, bridging understanding, and community cohesiveness. In terms of addressing trauma at the individual level, narratives have been shown to encourage healing, empowerment, and a greater sense of self, even when communities are suffering from the effects of complex trauma (Cox, 2000; Mamon et al., 2017; Monk et al., 1997; Parry & Doan, 1994; Sunwolf, 1999). This is particularly important to the Black residents of the northern part of the city, whose narratives have not been told from their viewpoints or taken into consideration with much of the local policy around law enforcement, economic development, education, and health.

In November 2017, we began a series called Community Conversations through Assisi House, Inc. These conversations were funded by the Interdisciplinary Research Leadership (IRL) Program through the Robert Wood Johnson Foundation (RWJF). Community Conversations were community dialogues where small groups of residents (N = 66) convened to share their narratives inspired by their perceptions about the links among health, race, space, and place. Using restorative justice as an overarching vision for the city, we began with small-scale meetings and narrative sharing. We created a safe space for the sharing of emotion and allowed follow-up discussions to lead toward understanding and agreement among participants where it was possible.

Conversations were held in three different sections of the city: the northern part of the city, the central section of the city, and the southern part of the city. In each case, meetings were free and open to the public and in places easily accessible by public transportation and with ample parking. Participants were recruited through social media, television announcements, radio announcements, and door-to-door canvassing. Participants were asked a series of discussion prompts in an open forum, and afterward were invited to complete follow-up questions and to share their stories for use in other forums and community gatherings.

We also interviewed policymakers one-on-one with the same prompts. We focused on collecting their stories as we did with residents (N = 6). We conducted interviews with the mayor, city councilpersons, and the chief health policymaking officer for the City-Parish of Baton Rouge. Interviews were conducted in April 2018.

We provided to community members and policymakers these prompts around health and housing:

What do you like best about living in this community?
What does being healthy mean to you?

Describe a healthy home.

Describe a healthy community.

What link do you see between health and housing?

What role, if any at all, does race play in health and housing in this community?

What should be known about your community that isn't widely known?

In all cases, we gave impromptu follow-up prompts as discussions went on, we provided structured demographic surveys for participants to complete, and we invited them to share even more of their stories with us via phone, video conferencing, email, or video recording.

The Community Conversation series overall included seventy-six participants, with 89.5 percent of participants identifying as Black, 9.2 percent of participants identifying as White, and 1.31 percent identifying as Hispanic or Latino. The sample was overwhelmingly female with nine of every ten participants identifying as female and 10 percent identifying as male. The mean age was forty-one years of age, and the median age was thirty-three. The age groups with the most representation were twenty-two to twenty-six and fifty to sixty. The city was well-represented geographically with twenty-three zip codes reported from participants. Though all residents were impacted by the flood, either caring for flooded family members, experiencing a flooded workplace, or knowing someone who actually flooded, 40 percent of Community Conversation respondents' homes were flooded, while 60 percent reported not personally suffering flooding of their homes.

The two zip codes most heavily represented at Community Conversations were 70814 and 70816. These zip codes represent clearly the racial divide in the city. The zip code 70814 is predominantly Black with just over 14,000 residents. It is located in the northern section of the city. Zip code 70816 has well over twice the population of 70814, but is predominantly White and located in the southern part of the city.

In the community discussion, notions of health took on a completely different connotation than policymakers imagined. While community members spoke of economic well-being through jobs, positive interactions with neighbors, improved educational opportunities, a living wage, and access to healthcare, policymakers spoke of regulations, such as yards being mowed, proper connections for mobile homes, and ensuring trash was picked up. This disconnect gives us clues that residents and policymakers are not speaking the same language when it comes to health outcomes.

Race, as expected, was more complicated in our discussions. Generally speaking, Black community residents across both zip codes shared narratives that reflected the inequalities in Baton Rouge, whether it was police brutality or the desire for better public schools and more job opportunities. Both Black and White residents talked about wanting more safety and more jobs, but White residents did not realize or recognize the needs of their Black counterparts. Instead they wondered about how individual family structure, educational levels, and parenting practices affected those suffering from inequality. Both groups expressed a desire to see the city get healthier and for Louisiana to move from the bottom of health and housing indicators to the top. Both groups expressed a desire to see Baton Rouge grow and provide opportunities for future generations and to have more businesses and more amenities for everyone.

From our viewpoint, those who are suffering the most from the effects of racism and division were still not significantly represented in the Community Conversation series. There is also a disconnect with who was represented in Community Conversations in terms of citizens. Residents of both 70814 and 70816 have incomes higher than the average income in the city, and both populations are more likely to have high school diplomas and at least some college attendance. Residents who bear the brunt of policymaking or who are the intended beneficiaries of community programming were not fully represented. Further, many residents, both Black and White, with the power to make change were underrepresented as well. Nevertheless, the implications of the stories told in the conversations did lead to an important conclusion for the series. Increasing participation of community members in determining what will work in their own communities is vital to improving public health outcomes in Baton Rouge. Baton Rouge is a city polarized by racism. But is it also a city that has survived a summer that threatened to create dangerous and violent outcomes. As the city continues to rebuild itself those seeking to overcome the deep chasm of racism still have much work to do. As for our research, we are expanding our work to include unheard voices and stories that cut across race and lived experiences. We hope to make an impact as we seek to unite two communities into one thriving city.

Historical trauma is rarely directly acknowledged in local policymaking circles in Baton Rouge. Even within the context of addressing the needs of the local community, it would behoove Baton Rouge's policymakers to recognize the impact of policies that worsen historical trauma and also that perpetuate complex trauma. The city would greatly benefit if those in power would use the recognition of the effects of such traumas as a further reason to solicit the perspectives of marginalized groups in the policies that affect them so that the cycle of disempowerment and repeated trauma can be broken.

References

Bartlett, J. D., Griffin, J. L., Spinazzola, J., Fraser, J. G., Rosa Noroña, C., Bodian, R., Todd, M., Montagna, C., & Barto, B. (2018). The impact of a statewide trauma-informed care initiative in child welfare on the well-being of children and youth with complex trauma. *Children and Youth Services Review, 84,* 110–117.

Baton Rouge Area Foundation. (2016). *City stats guide: 2016.* Retrieved August 2, 2021, from https://static1.squarespace.com/static/564b4eabe4bod6f83cf45269/t/57a10efee6f2e1fc871e5aee/1470172931264/CItyStats+2016_WEB_SMALL.pdf

Berube, A., & Holmes, N. (2016, July 14). Minority under-representation in city and suburban policing. *The Avenue.* Retrieved August 2, 2021, from https://www.brookings.edu/blog/the-avenue/2016/07/14/minority-under-representation-in-city-and-suburban-policing/

Brown, D. W. (2016, July 18) The unsolved violence of Baton Rouge. *The Atlantic.* Retrieved August 2, 2021, from https://www.theatlantic.com/politics/archive/2016/07/protests-police-shooting-baton-rouge/491714/

Citydata.com. (2016). *Baton Rouge, LA.* Retrieved August 2, 2021, from http://www.city-data.com/city/Baton-Rouge-Louisiana.html

Cooper, F. R. (2020). Cop fragility and Blue Lives Matter. *University of Illinois Law Review, 621.* Retrieved August 2, 2021, from https://www.illinoislawreview.org/print/vol-2020-no-2/cop-fragility-and-blue-lives-matter/

Cox, J. H. (2000). "All this water imagery must mean something": Thomas King' revisions of narratives of domination and conquest in "Green Grass, Running Water." *American Indian Quarterly, 24*(2), 219–246.

Danieli, Y. (Ed.). 1998. *International handbook of multigenerational legacies of trauma.* Plenum Press.

DataUSA. (2017). *Baton Rouge, LA.* Retrieved August 2, 2021, from https://datausa.io/profile/geo/baton-rouge-la/#demographics

Deslatte, M. (2016, July 11). Long divided: Baton Rouge race relations under new scrutiny. *AP News.* Retrieved from https://www.apnews.com/72b1d5c37dde40459e53bcc1bb8f7a9a

Fausset, R., J. Turketwiz, J., & Blinder, A. (2016, July 18). In Baton Rouge a divided city faces two tragedies. *New York Times.* Retrieved August 2, 2021, from https://www.nytimes.com/2016/07/20/us/in-baton-rouge-a-divided-city-faces-two-different-tragedies.html

Frank, R. H., & Cook, P. J. (2010). *The winner-take-all society: Why the few at the top get so much more than the rest of us.* Random House.

Gallo, A. (2018, April 4). Despite missteps in push to move Baton Rouge Zoo, BREC board still backing Carolyn McKnight. *The Advocate.* Retrieved August 2, 2021, from http://www.theadvocate.com/baton_rouge/news/article_03f31166–3824-11e8 –8e04–5fc189b2cf93.html

Gallo, A., & Russell, G. (2016, August 9). Sobering stats: 110,000 homes worth $20B in flood-affected areas in Baton Rouge region, analysis says. *The Advocate.* Retrieved August 2, 2021, from http://www.theadvocate.com/louisiana_flood_2016/ article_62b54a48–662a-11e6-aade-afd357ccc11f.html

Harris, A. (2019, May 20). The new secession. *The Atlantic.* Retrieved August 2, 2021, from https://www.theatlantic.com/education/archive/2019/05/resegrega tion-baton-rouge-public-schools/589381/

Krieger, N. (2001). Theories for social epidemiology in the 21st century: An ecosocial perspective. *International Journal of Epidemiology, 30*(4), 668–677.

Louisiana Network. (2017, July 25). New Orleans, Baton Rouge among most segregated cities in country. KPEL965.com. Retrieved August 2, 2021, from https://kpel965 .com/new-orleans-baton-rouge-among-most-segregated-cities-in-country/

Mamon, D., McDonald, E. C., Lambert, J. F., & Cameron, A. Y. (2017). Using storytelling to heal trauma and bridge the cultural divide between veterans and civilians. *Journal of Loss and Trauma, 22*(8), 669–680.

Mancini, J. A., & Bowen, G. L. (2009). Community resilience: A social organization theory of action and change. In J. A. Mancini & K. A. Roberto (Eds.), *Pathways of human development: Explorations of change* (pp. 245–265). Lexington Books.

Mental Health America. (2018). Ranking the states 2018. *Mental Health America.* Retrieved March 30, 2018, from https://www.mhanational.org/issues/ranking -states-2018–0.

Mohatt, N. V., Thompson, A. B., Thai, N. D., and Tebes, J. K. (2014). Historical trauma as public narrative: A conceptual review of how history impacts present-day health. *Social Science & Medicine, 106*, 128–136.

Monk, G. E., Winslade, J. E., Crocket, K. E., & Epston, D. E. (1997). *Narrative therapy in practice: The archaeology of hope.* Jossey-Bass.

Parry, A., & Doan, R. E. (1994). *Story re-visions: Narrative therapy in the postmodern world.* Guilford Press.

Pettus-Davis, C., Veeh, C. A., Davis, M., & Tripodi, S. (2018). Gender differences in experiences of social support among men and women releasing from prison. *Journal of Social and Personal Relationships, 35*(9), 1161–1182.

Pinderhughes, H., Davis, R., & Williams, M. (2015). *Adverse community experiences and resilience: A framework for addressing and preventing community trauma.* Prevention Institute. Retrieved August 2, 2021, from https://www.preventioninstitute.org/sites/default/files/publications/Adverse%20Community%20Experiences%20and%20Resilience.pdf

Roberts, D. E. (2003). The social and moral cost of mass incarceration in African American communities. *Stanford Law Review, 56,* 1271.

Schulz, A., & Northridge, M. E. (2004). Social determinants of health: implications for environmental health promotion. *Health Education & Behavior, 31*(4), 455–471.

Sotero, M. (2006). A conceptual model of historical trauma: Implications for public health practice and research. *Journal of Health Disparities Research and Practice, 1*(1), 93–108.

Sunwolf. (1999). The pedagogical and persuasive effects of Native American lesson stories, Sufi wisdom tales, and African dilemma tales. *Howard Journal of Communication, 10*(1), 47–71.

Van Ness, D., & Strong, K. H. (2003). *Inclusion.* Anderson Publishing.

Vera Institute of Justice. (2015, December 15). *Incarceration trends.* https://www.vera.org/projects/incarceration-trends

Yehuda, R., Bell, A., Bierer, L. M., & Schmeidler, J. (2008). Maternal, not paternal, PTSD is related to increased risk for PTSD in offspring of Holocaust survivors. *Journal of Psychiatric Research, 42*(13), 1104–1111.

Yehuda, R., Cai, G., Golier, J. A., Sarapas, C., Galea, S., Ising, M., Rein, T., Schmeidler, J., Müller-Myhsok, B., Holsboer, F., & Buxbaum, J. D. (2009). Gene expression patterns associated with posttraumatic stress disorder following exposure to the World Trade Center attacks. *Biological Psychiatry, 66*(7), 708–711.

Yehuda, R., Daskalakis, N. P., Bierer, L. M., Bader, H. N., Klengel, T., Holsboer, F., & Binder, E. B. (2016). Holocaust exposure induced intergenerational effects on FKBP5 methylation. *Biological Psychiatry, 80*(5), 372–380.

Yehuda, R., Daskalakis, N. P., Lehrner, A., Desarnaud, F., Bader, H. N., Makotkine, I., Flory, J. D., Bierer, L. M., & Meaney, M. J. (2014). Influences of maternal and paternal PTSD on epigenetic regulation of the glucocorticoid receptor gene in Holocaust survivor offspring. *American Journal of Psychiatry 171*(8), 872–880.

Yehuda, R., & LeDoux, J. (2007). Response variation following trauma: A translational neuroscience approach to understanding PTSD. *Neuron, 56*(1), 19–32.

Chapter 4

Increasing Housing Stability

Benefits and Challenges of Partnering with a Policy Advocate on Research to Inform Policy and Practice

Mina Silberberg, Donna J. Biederman, and Emily Carmody

The partnership described in this chapter was based on the team members' shared belief that all people deserve a home. At the same time, our individual contributions were shaped by distinct roles and perspectives. The initial impetus for the work came from two faculty at Duke—Mina Silberberg and Donna Biederman—but the research question itself came from an urgent practice–based concern brought to the research team by Emily Carmody, a project director at the North Carolina Coalition to End Homelessness. Silberberg—a political scientist who had worked in the fields of health policy and community health research/evaluation—was seeking opportunities to address social drivers of health. Biederman—a former emergency department nurse and case manager—had significant clinical, programmatic, and research experience focused on the health-related needs of people experiencing homelessness. This was her first opportunity to contribute to policymaking beyond the local level. Carmody had been advocating for the North Carolina Department of Health and Human Services to use Medicaid funding to finance tenancy support services (TSS), and the state had recently decided to do so. However, Carmody was concerned that a service definition created without benefit of knowledge about promising practices in the field could lead to poor TSS implementation and poor outcomes for the population being served, which could discredit TSS and restrict future funding.

The goal of our collaborative research project, therefore, was to provide information that could be used by state Medicaid offices, other financing/ regulatory bodies, and service providers to make TSS both widely available and highly effective in the new funding environment. We were also interested in the role that health services and health-related goals might play in TSS provision and regulation.

The experience of conducting and disseminating our research findings confirmed our initial belief that interdisciplinary community-engaged research (ICEnR) with leadership from a policy advocate and researchers had great potential for generating information to inform regulatory design. The regulations by which policy is operationalized are crucial to policy effectiveness, but there are significant barriers to the translation of research into regulatory practice. While ICEnR addresses many barriers to translation, there are few prior examples in the literature of using it to inform regulation, particularly with an advocate as a team member. Benefits of this ICEnR approach for our team included Carmody's existing relationships with stakeholders and specialized knowledge of the regulatory domain, process, and context; and her enhanced visibility as part of the team. Challenges of the approach were conflicting time demands, differing goals of team members, risks to Carmody's professional relationships if stakeholders were unhappy with our process or product, and concerns from one stakeholder group about sharing data with a policy advocate. We recommend to others three strategies that helped us to address these challenges and optimize the benefits from our collaboration. First, Carmody was compensated for the same amount of time as Silberberg and Biederman. Second, the team engaged early in discussions of motivations, expectations, and fears. Third, proactive attention was given to the advantages and risks of Carmody's role in the policy domain.

Conducting regulatory research is challenging, requiring highly detailed knowledge of the subject matter and design options, and the implications of these options for those affected by the regulation. Moreover, there are multiple obstacles to the translation of study findings into action. This chapter presents a case study of interdisciplinary community-engaged research (ICEnR)—the process of researchers and community members co-creating knowledge—conducted by the authors to generate evidence for a Medicaid tenancy support service (TSS) definition. We argue that our approach—involving a policy advocate as an investigator and engaging a wide swath of impacted community stakeholders including TSS clients, state leadership, state agency staff, and TSS providers—has helped our team address the challenges of regulatory research.[1]

The chapter begins with background on TSS and the importance of regulatory research in this area. We then describe community engagement and its relatively untapped potential for the study of regulation. This background is followed by our case description, explaining the impetus for our work together and its trajectory. The subsequent discussion section highlights lessons learned from our experience about the benefits of ICEnR—in particular, the inclusion of an advocate—on regulatory research, the challenges of this approach, and actions that can address those challenges to facilitate a successful outcome.

---

1. Throughout this chapter the term "regulatory research" is used to encompass both rules as informal administrative conventions and regulations as formal requirements.

Background

Institutionalization, Homelessness, and Health

There is an enormous need in the United States to help individuals who are institutionalized or experiencing homelessness obtain homes in the community. In 1999, the United States Supreme Court held in *Olmstead v. L.C.* that unjustified segregation of persons with disabilities constituted discrimination in violation of the Americans with Disabilities Act (DOJ, n.d.), thereby codifying the importance of community-based housing. Yet, almost two decades later, there are thousands of people with physical, mental, and developmental disabilities unnecessarily living in institutionalized settings. In North Carolina alone, the Department of Justice estimated in 2011 that 5,800 individuals with mental illness resided in institutions known as adult care home facilities (Perez, 2011).

At the same time, more than half a million Americans were identified as experiencing homelessness on one night (i.e., sleeping outside or in emergency shelters, or residing in transitional housing) in 2018 (U.S. Department of Housing and Urban Development [HUD], 2018). Of those, an estimated 96,913, or 17.5 percent, were identified as experiencing chronic homelessness and therefore likely to benefit from affordable housing with support services (HUD, 2018). Research has demonstrated that homelessness contributes to poor physical and mental health and health services outcomes, and to higher rates of mortality (Castellow, Kloos, & Townley, 2015; Morrison, 2009; Oppenheimer, Nurius, & Green, 2016; Shalen, 2017).

Permanent Supportive Housing as a Policy Solution

One of the most promising policy solutions for decreasing institution-alization and homelessness is moving people into community housing using a model known as permanent supportive housing. Permanent supportive housing combines long-term affordable housing and tenancy support services (TSS), broadly defined as assistance with obtaining and maintaining a home. TSS can include anything from helping with a housing application to solving hygiene problems that could result in eviction to connecting a consumer with health services. Research shows that permanent supportive housing is associated with decreased homelessness and increased housing tenure (Benston, 2015; Burt, 2012; Byrne et al., 2014; Henwood, Katz, & Gilmer, 2015; Rog et al., 2014). Research also shows an association between permanent supportive housing and positive health outcomes, including decreased alcohol use, improved HIV status, decreased use of acute health services, and increased use of outpatient services (Buchanan et al., 2009; Collins et al., 2012; Mackelprang, Collins, & Clifasefi, 2014; Martinez & Burt, 2006; Rieke et al., 2015; Rog et al., 2014). A recent report noted that the evidentiary base demonstrating a causal relationship between permanent supportive housing and health outcomes is limited by inconsistencies in the definition of permanent supportive housing, lack of consensus on minimum standards for services, and poor data systems. Nonetheless, the report indicated that housing improves health and that permanent supportive housing helps a subset of people to obtain and maintain housing (National Academies of Sciences, Engineering, and Medicine, 2018).

Public financial support for permanent supportive housing has historically been limited, with funding coming primarily through the U.S. Department of Housing and Urban Development (HUD). However, on June 26, 2015, the Centers for Medicare and Medicaid Services (CMS) issued an informational bulletin advising that Medicaid funds could be used by states to reimburse for TSS (Wachino, 2015). While the bulletin reviewed mechanisms and gave examples of how states can use Medicaid to fund TSS, it left the implementation and regulation development, including waiver applications and service definitions, up to each state's Medicaid program. To utilize Medicaid funds for TSS, state Medicaid programs need to understand what successful TSS provision looks like and what regulatory environment supports effective TSS provision.

Research-Informed Regulation

The CMS decision to fund TSS is part of a larger shift toward addressing social drivers of health (SDoH) through Medicaid, reflected in new initiatives like the State Innovation Models that test new payment and service delivery options aimed at lowering costs while improving or maintaining quality of care. Medicaid officials now find themselves in the position of funding—and therefore overseeing—services that do not necessarily fit healthcare regulatory models.

The expansion of Medicaid into SDoH increases the importance of using research to inform new regulations. However, there are obstacles to the translation of research into human services policy (Macoubrie & Harrison, 2013). Often agencies and individuals with the greatest knowledge of the details of regulation and the greatest interest in this type of research—particularly those on the front lines of regulation—lack the time, expertise, or other resources necessary for conducting research or translating it into action. At the same time, academic researchers are often drawn toward the knowledge generation and peer-reviewed publications that are rewarded in their institutions and away from issues of policy and practice (Macoubrie & Harrison, 2013). In addition, research often takes a long time to complete, while policy decisions are on a short timeline. Translation of research also requires an in-depth understanding of the implications of a particular context; researchers may lack that contextual understanding, while practitioners may understand the context, but lack the means to conduct research to affect policy change. These challenges to the creation and translation of policy research are compounded for regulatory research, which requires interest in and knowledge of detailed policy issues and their relationship to specific policy contexts. Researcher engagement with policy advocates may help surmount many of these barriers.

Community-Engaged Research

Community engagement has been described as "the process of working collaboratively with and through groups of people affiliated by geographic proximity, special interest, or similar situations to address issues affecting the well-being of those people" (Centers for Disease Control and Prevention [CDC], 1997, p. 9). While emphasizing the importance of engaging communities, who it is hoped will benefit from change, engagement approaches have also been used to engage a wide variety of stakeholders, for example, service providers, funders, etc. Engagement has been promoted by scholars and funders because of evidence of multiple benefits. It fosters relationships of trust between researchers and practitioners; increases the relevance of research questions and the ways in which findings are presented to stakeholders; improves research quality through community assistance with recruitment, instrument design, interpretation of results, and other support of the research process; and facilitates direct benefit from research to communities in the form of compensation for their time, sharing of knowledge, and demystification of the research process (Staley, 2009; Viswanathan et al., 2004). Engagement also encourages development of interventions that are tailored to the local context, creates a common language for researchers and community members, focuses on sustainable change, and strengthens the likelihood that research can and will be used to inform action (Wallerstein & Duran, 2017).

Engagement varies in philosophy and strategy. Wallerstein and Duran (2017) have conceptualized a continuum of participatory or engaged research. On one end of the continuum is Kurt Lewin's "action research" approach, which gives primacy to the benefits of engaged research for practical problem solving. On the other end is "liberation" research, in the spirit of the work of Paolo Freire, that encourages marginalized groups to use action and reflection to develop their own understanding of and take action on the conditions oppressing them.

Engagement has most often been used to promote and inform two types of action. The first is community-level change. This type of engagement generally emphasizes engagement with community members who are direct beneficiaries of the hoped-for changes and can be placed at or near the Freirian end of the continuum. A second, less common, approach to engagement addresses broad policy concerns, whether from a Lewinian problem-solving perspective, a Freirian liberation perspective, or a combination of the two.

Engagement to address regulatory research is much less common than either of the two types of research just described. Rarer still is the engagement of a policy advocate toward this end. The case study presented here describes a two-tiered engagement model—an approach on the Lewinian end of the engagement continuum—in which a homelessness services advocate works with two trained researchers as a fully co-equal research leader, while TSS service providers, government agencies, and consumers inform the study in more limited ways.

Case Description
Forming the Team

In the spring of 2016, two of the authors, Mina Silberberg and Donna Biederman, came together to answer the Robert Wood Johnson Foundation (RWJF)'s Interdisciplinary Research Leaders (IRL) call for proposals. Silberberg has a doctorate in political science and postdoctoral training in health policy and health services research. She is a faculty member in the Department of Family Medicine and Community Health in Duke Medical School and has worked in the field of health policy and community health research and evaluation for over two decades. Biederman, a former emergency department nurse and case manager for persons experiencing homelessness, is a faculty member in the Duke University School of Nursing. She had conducted several research studies with individuals experiencing homelessness, was an active member of the National Health Care for the Homeless Council's Respite Care Providers Network steering committee, and a co–primary investigator on a Hillman Innovations in Care grant to develop a transitional care program for persons with a medical issue exiting an institutional setting (e.g., hospital, behavioral health facility, jail) without a home.

Biederman identified Emily Carmody, a program director with the North Carolina Coalition to End Homelessness (NCCEH), as a potential partner. Carmody had vast knowledge of homelessness, housing policy, and issues specific to the state from her past work in the field as a case manager and her current role as a policy advocate, and she had served as an expert on regional and state homelessness during the Hillman grant site visit.

Despite her passion for issues of housing and homelessness, it would have been impossible for Carmody to take any significant amount of time away from her job to conduct work that was not critical to the mission of her agency. However, through its grant program, RWJF provided the same stipend for the community partner's time—intended to cover approximately one day of work per week—that it provided each researcher. Moreover, the researchers agreed to work on an issue that Carmody saw as critical to her agency—specifically generating data that could inform Medicaid funding for TSS.

For seven years, NCCEH had advocated for the North Carolina Department of Health and Human Services (NC DHHS) to use Medicaid funding to finance TSS. The state had recently agreed. However, as with many advocacy efforts, the win came with a new set of challenges. There were still many decisions to be made about the specific Medicaid vehicle (e.g., 1115 waiver, rehabilitation services) used to fund TSS and other elements of the service definition. Medicaid service definitions describe what services can be reimbursed and address funding details such as participant eligibility requirements, the specifics of covered services, and reimbursement rates.

Carmody was concerned that a service definition created without benefit of knowledge about promising practices in the field could lead to poor TSS implementation and poor outcomes for the population being served, which could discredit TSS and restrict future funding. She also knew that, faced with large workloads and looming deadlines, state officials rarely had time to read research literature that might inform regulatory development. Moreover, the literature on TSS she had encountered did not address the questions of front-line practice and its regulation that she saw as most relevant to the service definition. She was deeply invested in the question of how Medicaid funding could be most effectively used. In fact, this was the only research topic on which she was interested in working.

Defining the Research Question

Silberberg and Biederman understood the need to turn the goal of informing Medicaid regulation into research questions that were precise, feasible to answer, and assumed no a priori answers.[2] Together, drawing on their diverse expertise, the team formulated four research questions that formed the basis for the study:

1.   What constitutes TSS effectiveness (i.e., what do stakeholders perceive to be the key outcomes of supportive housing and quality TSS)? Is improved health one of those outcomes?

2.   What are the promising practices of effective TSS providers?

3.   Which aspects of provider agency context support effective TSS that is responsive to client needs and accessible to a diverse population? Which create challenges?

4.   Which aspects of local, state, and federal regulation support the delivery of effective TSS that is responsive to client needs and accessible to a diverse population? Which create challenges?

The research team brought their varied expertise to the formulation of these questions. The overarching research question of how to provide,

2. The team members share a belief that no person is completely neutral. Throughout the course of the project, they used strategies primarily derived from research training to try to recognize their biases and assumptions and to maximize their openness to new ways of understanding the issues being studied. For example, qualitative data collection was purposefully preceded by a discussion of assumptions.

fund, and regulate tenancy support services came from Carmody's work as both a service provider and a policy advocate. Silberberg's background in program evaluation and public administration made her attentive to the role of context in shaping the outcomes of service provision and funding. Biederman, with her experience with health and healthcare for persons experiencing homelessness, reminded the team at this stage and throughout the project of the varied implications of homelessness and housing for health.

Developing the Study Design

Through collaborative deliberation, the team arrived at a mixed-methods design employing comparative case studies (which in turn employed document review, interviews, and focus groups), key participant interviews, and quantitative secondary data analysis. Biederman and Silberberg felt that qualitative research on the state context and case studies of provider agencies was a good approach to answering the research questions, given the strengths of these approaches for facilitating the development of new conceptual frameworks in relatively uncharted territory. Because the grant period was short, the researchers suggested limiting the number of cases. Based on their knowledge of case study methods, they suggested that the cases studied should be "diverse"—varying on important dimensions—and "extreme," that is, representing highly effective TSS provision (Seawright & Gerring, 2008).

In selecting the cases, Carmody's knowledge of the field was crucial. She understood that the cases would need to represent the two very different types of agencies that provide TSS in North Carolina—agencies dedicated to housing people experiencing homelessness and agencies providing mental health and related services. This variable of agency type was the primary dimension on which the case studies would be "diverse." Furthermore, Carmody could immediately identify a successful agency of each type: (1) Homeward Bound, in Asheville, North Carolina, an organization dedicated to housing the homeless that had an 89 percent success rate for obtaining housing for clients within two years and maintaining them in housing for at least six months, a HUD performance benchmark, and was credited with reducing chronic homelessness in its county by 58 percent; and (2) the University of North Carolina Center for Excellence in Community Mental Health, which had been chosen by NC DHHS to provide training on the Assertive Community Treatment team model of service provision because of its success in this area. Assertive Community Treatment, a community-based approach that provides supports at a level usually found only in-patient settings, is one of the key mechanisms through which mental health agencies currently provide TSS. In addition to being "extreme" in their performance and diverse in agency type, these two agencies were diverse in geographic location. The team decided to use a combination of encounter and administrative data and interviews/ focus groups with service providers, consumers, and landlords for the case studies.

In addition to the case studies, the study design had two other components: analysis of existing state-level data, and qualitative research with state officials. Carmody was well-acquainted with and suggested use of the Homelessness Management Information System (HMIS), which stores data elements collected by homeless service agencies in the community, including all such agencies receiving HUD funding. These data could be used to determine overall outcomes for homeless service agencies that provide permanent supportive housing in the state, make comparisons of those outcomes to those of the case study agencies, and analyze how outcomes varied by consumer characteristics. Interviews with officials from NC DHHS and housing specialists from the regional managed care organizations (MCOs) that administer safety-net mental health services would provide data across all four research questions.

At a later stage, the team decided that time and resources allowed for research into what could be learned from a state already using Medicaid funding for TSS. Carmody suggested Louisiana because of the similarities to North Carolina in geography, political climate, and Medicaid systems. Experts on Medicaid and homelessness confirmed this choice, and we added interviews with Louisiana state officials and the directors of two high-performing permanent supportive housing agencies there to our study.

Engaging Stakeholders

Our initial request of stakeholders was an endorsement of our research proposal. With Carmody's knowledge of and relationships with key organizations, thirteen stakeholders wrote letters of support for our grant, including the NC DHHS Medicaid Office, the provider agencies we would be studying, and the MCOs. Quarterly meetings with NC DHHS and our two provider agencies were invaluable for fleshing out our research design (e.g., identifying the sample) and plans.

As part of our engagement strategy, we also formed a consumer advisory council made up of permanent supportive housing program participants. Carmody's contacts with a local housing agency and the area MCO allowed for potential consumer advisory council members to be identified and contacted quickly. We invited eight individuals to the consumer advisory council and ended up with a group of three members who consistently participated in meetings.

Increasing Team Cohesion

As the team moved forward on detailing the study plan and design, we also participated in team-building exercises required by the IRL program. These included conversations about what motivated each of us to engage in housing research, our fears and concerns about the work, our expectations of each other, and our work styles; creation of a "communication covenant"; discussion of hypothetical case scenarios of common research challenges; and development of a shared team history. Three revelations that emerged from this work were particularly important in strengthening team bonds. First, we learned that, while our paths and specific experiences had been different, each of us had at some point worked directly with low-income communities, whether as a community organizer, social worker, or healthcare professional. Second, Carmody explained that, by building on her relationships with state agencies and service providers for the work of this project, she was putting those relationships at risk if this project was perceived to be unsuccessful or controversial. This expression of vulnerability impressed on the researchers the importance of striving for transparency with community partners at all times and solidified our commitment to producing research that would be both rigorous and useful.

Third, these exercises generated a discussion of the possibility that our research findings would contradict previously held beliefs. This was especially important for Carmody, who had passionately invested in promoting the policies she and her agency believed to be beneficial to people experiencing homelessness and previously institutionalized. It was possible, for example, that our interview and focus group participants would see minimal value in TSS. Carmody proactively asserted that the mission of her agency is to support practices that help individuals to live independently in the community; indications of TSS ineffectiveness would require the agency to reconsider its positions. The discussion reinforced for the researchers the importance of rigor and sensitivity in their work. For the advocate, the discussion provided insight into the challenge of remaining unbiased. Bringing awareness to these issues laid the groundwork for the team to continue to discuss them as the study progressed.

Determining Study Participants, Developing Instruments, and Planning Data Collection

As we moved ahead to select study participants, Biederman and Silberberg brought their understanding of the format and objectives of focus groups and interviews to the discussion. Carmody's knowledge of roles at service provider agencies and the state government was important in defining the participant list and which participants should be interviewed (because of the uniqueness of their roles or experience or the need for confidentiality) and which included in focus groups (because of the potential for dynamic discussion of similar and different perspectives). Ultimately, participants included administrators, managers, and front-line staff at the two NC case study agencies, agency clients, and landlords/property managers associated with the properties where those clients live; state officials in both North Carolina and Louisiana; and housing specialists at the NC MCOs and the executive directors of two well-regarded provider agencies in Louisiana. Input from the consumer advisory council was particularly important in highlighting the importance of the triangular relationship among consumers, service providers, and landlords—an insight that led us to include landlords among our respondents.

Focus group and interview instruments for use with these respondents were designed to obtain perspectives on perceived outcomes of TSS, promising practices, contextual facilitators and barriers to effective practice (including, but not limited to the regulatory environment), and issues associated with Medicaid funding for TSS. As we developed those instruments, Carmody provided insights into the specific issues of concern to the state officials related to funding TSS though Medicaid and provider agencies we hoped to influence, the language that spoke to our different stakeholder groups, and the topics our study participants could address. Her understanding of the needs and concerns of state officials, MCOs, and provider agencies provided the team with a starting point for discussion with these stakeholders when we approached them for their input into study planning and design. For example, having learned that the Medicaid office is particularly concerned about how best to set payment rates and train staff, we focused on those issues in data collection. The consumer advisory council was particularly helpful with the wording of the consumer focus group instrument and provided the idea to include landlords as study participants.

Data Collection

Early on, we adjusted data collection plans. Through Carmody's engagement with them, we learned that NC DHHS staff began developing their service definition almost at the same time we began our research. With no research findings to share but wishing to be of assistance, we arranged two meetings between NC DHHS and the Louisiana Department of Health, with experts on housing and Medicaid in attendance. These meetings provided NC DHHS with useful information, generated data for us, and strengthened our relationship with them.

From there, we moved on to our study as designed. Stakeholder engagement facilitated aspects of qualitative data collection. Notably, the NC provider agencies helped schedule our interviews and focus groups with their personnel, consumers, and landlords—something we thought we would have to do ourselves, potentially with less success and certainly more slowly than the agencies were able to do it. Interviews and focus groups were conducted by the research team in pairs to reduce the potential impact of individual bias. One member of the team led the discussion while the other managed the audio recording equipment and took backup notes.

Inclusion of an advocate on the team was a double-edged sword for data collection. We recognized that, given competition among the state's MCOs and broader political controversies about their role in the mental health system, having a policy advocate present during focus groups with MCO housing specialists could suppress honest conversation. Carmody therefore spearheaded team outreach to the housing specialists, whom she knew professionally, but was not involved in the focus groups themselves.

For secondary data collection, Carmody's experience working with HMIS and general knowledge of provider agency data systems accelerated our discussions with the providers and HMIS lead agency about their secondary data and the development of data-sharing agreements. However, to actually obtain data from HMIS, we needed approval of the repository Governance Committee, made up of representatives from each of the state's Continuums of Care (CoC) (regional planning bodies for homelessness services), some of whom expressed a concern that Carmody might draw conclusions from the data about differences in outcomes by region or agency. As a result, receipt of the data was stalled for a year. At the same time, Carmody's awareness of CoC sensitivities facilitated negotiations. We agreed to provide agencies with the opportunity to opt out of the data set (only a few did) and restrict data access to the university researchers, and researchers were provided with a data set that was deidentified at the individual, program, and CoC levels.

Data Analysis

The benefits of having a team that were both community-engaged and interdisciplinary were very apparent during data analysis. For the qualitative analysis, for example, Silberberg's experience with case study methodology provided a general analytic framework, while Biederman's strong training in qualitative methods helped the group to develop the details of a phased analytic approach that simultaneously allowed for collaboration, reliability, and insights from the team's diverse perspectives. The richness afforded by this diversity is apparent in what team members saw in the data. For example, Carmody was particularly sensitive to the differences in context and funding for mental health and homeless services agencies; Biederman was attuned to nuances in participants' responses and Silberberg to tradeoffs among regulatory goals. Community engagement in analysis extended beyond the research team. Several key findings were brought to the consumer advisory council for their reaction, which provided validation of the qualitative analysis, and the study agencies were each provided with their case study writeup for validation or "member-checking." Designing quantitative analysis also drew on the team's diverse expertise; for example, in making decisions about collapsing categories, Biederman and Silberberg could speak to their experience with statistical analysis, while Carmody made sure that new categories would represent groupings that were meaningful.

Translation of Research into Action

True to engagement principles, planning and laying the groundwork for translation were central to our work from the beginning. Carmody brought her knowledge of stakeholders and how they receive information, which included a one-day symposium for key stakeholders and a presentation at her agency's annual conference for service providers. Given the tight timeline state officials faced with their initial service definition, we began working to help them translate research into action earlier than planned. In addition to the conversation with the officials from Louisiana, we provided them with a summary of our review of the existing relevant literature.

Even before data analysis was complete, our engagement process developed relationships that have already had implications for our involvement in state policy. In spring of 2018, our NC DHHS contacts brought our work to the attention of the state health director and the staff who lead the state's new Healthy Opportunities program, designed to encourage payers and providers to address SDoH. As a result of the visibility the study gave her, Carmody was invited to join the committee developing a standard approach to assessment of needs related to SDoH and to another committee charged with drafting service definitions and rate-setting for services addressing SDoH. In addition, relationships with NC DHHS leadership resulted in the development of a new rehousing program in late summer 2018 in the wake of Hurricane Florence, Back@ Home, with the goal of helping families who were still in disaster shelters or staying in unsafe or unstable arrangements quickly transition to safe and sustainable longer-term housing.

The symposium at which we presented our summary findings was well attended, and included representatives of the agencies we studied,

Carmody's agency, several different divisions of NC DHHS, state officials from Louisiana, the consumer advisory council, and national experts on TSS. We designed the day to be interactive, creating the space for participants to actively think about the implications of our study for their work, and also provided opportunities for networking. Relationships were forged at the symposium that have led to peer agency bidirectional learning at the service provider and state agency levels as well as ongoing dialogue across sectors. Moreover, as a result of the symposium, we were invited to meet with a senior official at NC DHHS who, based on that conversation, subsequently modified the rollout of a revised Medicaid service definition that included TSS.

Lessons Learned

Regulatory research poses many challenges for study design and translation. The highly detailed nature of regulation requires both an intense subject matter expertise and an understanding of the relevant local, state, or national context in which regulation must be effectively formulated and implemented. At the same time, research in this area benefits from a wider awareness of relevant regulation from other contexts (see table 4.1).

The interdisciplinary nature of our team greatly benefited the regulatory research described here. Carmody is particularly expert in the housing field, Silberg in community health, and Biederman in the intersection of the two. As a practitioner of program evaluation and a student of public administration, Silberg was attentive to the role of context in the outcomes of service provision and funding and was trained in case study methods. Biederman brought to the project a strong understanding of the strengths and challenges of persons experiencing homelessness, particularly in regards to their health, and formal training

Table 4.1   Advocate Contributions to the Challenges of Regulatory Research

Regulatory research challenges	Advocate contributions
Highly detailed knowledge of regulation subject matter, design, process, and implications required	Advocate specialization allows for an understanding of the subject matter details needed for regulation design. Advocate understanding of regulatory process assists in translating research findings into regulatory recommendations.
Risk of research remaining siloed and not influencing regulation design or implementation	Advocate relationships with key staff at executive branch agencies provides access to regulation design process and allows for engagement of key staff in the research study. Advocate understanding of the challenges faced by staff in regulation design influences research questions and increases buy-in from the regulatory agency.
Regulation development follows a changing timeline that may not match study timelines	Advocate knowledge and monitoring of regulation development can inform study timeline, and if possible, team adjusts study timeline to maximize impact on regulation development. Advocate understanding of the larger implications of regulation development at the local, state, and federal levels provides multiple opportunities for research to influence regulation at design and implementation stages.
Knowledge of the specific context for regulation and broader knowledge of examples of similar regulation design required	Advocate specialization allows for an understanding of the context needed for regulation design. Advocate relationships with other states and advocacy organizations increases the ability to learn from other agencies with similar regulation and incorporate their experiences into the study.

in a variety of approaches to qualitative research. Carmody understood the language and conceptual models of social work, the discipline most closely aligned with TSS. This diversity of disciplinary perspectives and backgrounds contributed to the comprehensiveness and relevance of the research questions and the quality of data collection and analysis.

Even more striking than the interdisciplinary nature of the authors' work, however, is the impact of our community engagement approach, particularly the inclusion of a policy advocate as a coequal member of the research team. Understanding specific regulatory questions and options *and* the unique political circumstances and other contextual factors surrounding regulatory design in particular states or locales is challenging. Policy advocates are well positioned to help research teams overcome this challenge by harnessing their expertise to understand the history, context, and detailed concerns associated with the regulation they are attempting to influence. In the case study presented here, the inclusion of an advocate focused the team on a regulatory question of which they were not previously aware and helped identify the specific issues that would be of most importance to policymakers and key data sources, as well as a comparison state with a similar policy context. All through the study, she also alerted the team to political sensitivities.

As illustrated in this case study, drafting of regulations can present as a moving target. The changing timelines, document versions, and comment periods associated with this process may be daunting for researchers, especially when attempting to have an impact on regulation design that is in progress. A policy advocate who is familiar with the local regulatory process can aid researchers in tracking regulation changes and shifting their study design to achieve maximum impact.

Policy advocates also benefit research teams though their relationships with stakeholders, ranging from consumers, to service providers, to policymakers. In particular, state-level advocates regularly work with and can provide access to executive branch staff. Through these relationships, the team can better understand the questions that stakeholders have and thereby design studies that prove useful to these staff. Relationships also assist in research translation to ensure that study information does not remain siloed and instead affects regulatory design. Finally, policy advocates have relationships with other advocates who work on similar issues around the country. This network of advocates helps to inform research teams by providing a broader contextual view of what has been done or is being attempted in other places. Researchers are then able to provide both detailed recommendations and wider contextual background for stakeholders, which increases the likelihood that their study will influence regulatory design.

Despite the many benefits of having an advocate on a team, researchers must understand the inherent challenges of including these community members (see table 4.2). Advocates work to influence policymakers and regulatory design to achieve an outcome they see as beneficial. While researchers also bring their own preexisting beliefs to a study, our team's conversations reflected the significant investment of an advocate in the position that she has been promoting. Research teams need to recognize this potential conflict and create team norms that allow for ongoing discussion about it. Teams also need to incorporate measures to reduce the potential impact of all members' biases and the bias created by respondents' preexisting relationships with the advocate. The advocate must also understand from the outset the inherent risks to participating in a research study and account for the chances that the results of the study disprove her current policy stance. Our discussion resulted in consensus that if the data were to show something different than Carmody expected, that would only be to the good in strengthening her agency's ability to achieve its ultimate goal of promoting the well-being of people experiencing homelessness. Other risks associated with having an advocate on a research team pertain to the advocate's existing relationships. While having relationships with key staff, providers, and other advocates greatly benefits the team, research partners need to recognize there is an inherent risk to using these relationships for research purposes. If the study is viewed as a nuisance or unhelpful, the advocate's relationships could be damaged, which could impede her future work. Conversely, the advocate's previous challenging or negative relationships with stakeholders may create barriers to obtaining data or disseminating study

Table 4.2   Challenges and Facilitators of Advocate Research Participation

Challenges	Facilitators
Advocate's desire for research to validate platform and mission	Discuss at team formation inherent biases so that these can be identified and addressed throughout the study.
	Build an understanding of the inherent risks to the advocate's work by participating in research study.
Negative politics and relationships that surround advocate's work and decrease access to information and influence	Utilize the team approach by having research partners engage others who have a negative bias toward the advocate and address their concerns with the advocate's participation in the study.
Risk to advocate's relationships with stakeholders if research is perceived as unhelpful or a nuisance	Identify this risk at team formation and develop norms around engagement with stakeholders.
Advocate's investment of time in study decreases capacity of nonprofit agency	Provide direct financial compensation to the nonprofit agency to account for advocate's time.
	Engage the advocate in study design so that the research questions are mission-focused for the home agency.

results. In this case study, the advocate's candor about sensitivities relative to her agency facilitated negotiations over data acquisition from other stakeholders.

Advocates may not be able to dedicate large amounts of time to a research study. Many local policy advocates work for nonprofit agencies that cannot afford to use staff capacity for such activities. As in this case, researchers should involve policy advocates in the initial research design to ensure that the time spent on the study furthers the mission of the advocate's organization. By ensuring that the study is mission critical, buy-in from agency leadership is increased and adjustments can be made in current workloads to prioritize participating in the project. Teams also need to provide adequate financial compensation for the advocate's agency. While contracts with large university systems can prove burdensome for smaller nonprofit administrative staff, foundations that provide direct monetary compensation to agencies for staff participation may be more successful in bolstering advocate participation in research. Awareness of these issues enables researchers to create contexts where team participation appeals to advocates and their agencies.

Conclusion

The regulations by which policy is operationalized are crucial to policy effectiveness. This reality has become increasingly important as Medicaid expands to address housing and other SDoH that differ in nature from the direct medical care it was originally designed to support. However, there are significant barriers to the translation of research into regulatory practice, and, while engagement addresses many barriers to translation, it is not often used to inform regulation. The case study presented here illustrates the benefits of engaging a policy advocate on an interdisciplinary research team. These include the advocate's relationships with stakeholders and specialized knowledge of the regulatory domain, process, and context; and her enhanced visibility to policymakers as a member of the research team. The case study also illustrates challenges to advocate engagement, including time demands, differing goals, risks to advocate relationships, and the politicized nature of advocacy. Finally, the case study depicts strategies that address these challenges, including compensation for advocate time; early engagement; proactive discussions of motivations, expectations, and fears; and attention to the advocate's role in the policy domain.

Acknowledgments

A portion of this chapter appeared previously in Silberberg, M., Biederman, D.J., & Carmody, Emily. "Joining Forces: The Benefits and Challenges of Conducting Regulatory Research With a Policy Advocate." *Housing Policy Debate*, 29:3, (2019), 475–488, DOI: 10.1080/10511482.2018.1541923. Copyright © Virginia Polytechnic Institute and State University reprinted by permission of Taylor & Francis Ltd, http://www.tandfonline.com on behalf of Virginia Polytechnic Institute and State University.

References

Benston, E. A. (2015). Housing programs for homeless individuals with mental illness: Effects on housing and mental health outcomes. *Psychiatric Services, 66*(8), 806–816.

Buchanan, D., Kee, R., Sadowski, L. S., & Garcia, D. (2009). The health impact of supportive housing for HIV-positive homeless patients: A randomized controlled trial. *American Journal of Public Health, 99*(Suppl. 3), S675–680.

Burt, M. R. (2012). Impact of housing and work supports on outcomes for chronically homeless adults with mental illness: LA's HOPE. *Psychiatric Services, 63*(3), 209–215.

Byrne, T., Fargo, J. D., Montgomery, A. E., Munley, E., & Culhane, D. P. (2014). The relationship between community investment in permanent supportive housing and chronic homelessness. *Social Service Review, 88*(2), 234–263.

Castellow, J., Kloos, B., & Townley, G. (2015). Previous homelessness as a risk factor for recovery from serious mental illnesses. *Community Mental Health, 51*(6), 674–684.

Centers for Disease Control and Prevention (CDC). (1997). *Principles of community engagement* (1st ed.). CDC/ATSDR Committee on Community Engagement.

Collins, S. E., Clifasefi, S. L., Dana, E. A., Andrasik, M. P., Stahl, N., Kirouac, M., Welbaum, C., King, M., & Malone, D. K. (2012). Where harm reduction meets housing first: Exploring alcohol's role in a project-based housing first setting. *International Journal on Drug Policy, 23*(2), 111–119.

Henwood, B. F., Katz, M. L., & Gilmer, T. P. (2015). Aging in place within permanent supportive housing. *International Journal of Geriatric Psychiatry, 30*(1), 80–87.

Mackelprang, J. L., Collins, S. E., & Clifasefi, S. L. (2014). Housing First is associated with reduced use of emergency medical services. *Prehospital Emergency Care, 18*(4), 476–482.

Macoubrie, J., & Harrison, C. (2013, February). The value-added research dissemination framework. *OPRE Report* 2013–10.

Martinez, T. E., & Burt, M. R. (2006). Impact of permanent supportive housing on the use of acute care health services by homeless adults. *Psychiatric Services, 57*(7), 992–999.

Morrison, D. (2009). Homelessness as an independent risk factor for mortality: Results from a retrospective cohort study. *International Journal of Epidemiology, 38*(3), 877–883.

National Academies of Sciences, Engineering, and Medicine. (2018). *Permanent supportive housing: Evaluating the evidence for improving health outcomes among people experiencing chronic homelessness*. Washington, DC: National Academies Press. https://doi.org/10.17226/25133

Oppenheimer, S., Nurius, P., & Green, S. (2016). Homelessness history impacts on health outcomes and economic and risk behavior intermediaries: New insights from population data. *Journal of Contemporary Social Services, 97*(3), 230–242.

Perez, T. E. (2011, July 28). Letter to the Honorable Roy Cooper. Retrieved June 18, 2021, from https://www.ada.gov/olmstead/documents/nc_findings_letter.docx

Rieke, K., Smolsky, A., Bock, E., Erkes, L. P., Porterfield, E., & Watanabe-Galloway, S. (2015). Mental and nonmental health hospital admissions among chronically homeless adults before and after supportive housing placement. *Social Work in Public Health, 30*(6), 496–503.

Rog, D. J., Marshall, T., Dougherty, R. H., George, P., Daniels, A. S., Ghose, S. S., & Delphin-Rittmon, M. E. (2014). Permanent supportive housing: assessing the evidence. *Psychiatric Services, 65*(3), 287–294.

Seawright, J. & Gerring, J. (2008). Case selection techniques in case study research a menu of qualitative and quantitative options. *Political Research Quarterly, 61*(2), 294–308.

Shalen, E. (2017). Homelessness is an independent risk factor for cardiovascular disease hospital readmission in the California health care utilization project. *Circulation 135*(10).

Staley, K. (2009). *Exploring impact: Public involvement in NHS, public health, and social care research.* National Institutes for Health Research. Retrieved on June 18, 2021, from http://www.invo.org.uk/posttypepublication/exploring-impact -public-involvement-in-nhs-public-health-and-social-care-research/

U.S. Department of Housing and Urban Development (HUD). (2018). HUD 2018 continuum of care homeless assistance program homeless populations and subpopulations. Retrieved on June 18, 2021, from https://www.hudexchange .info/programs/coc/coc-homeless-populations-and-subpopulations-reports/

U.S. Department of Justice (DOJ). (n.d.). Information and technical assistance on the Americans with Disabilities Act. Retrieved June 10, 2018, from https://www .ada.gov/olmstead/olmstead_about.htm

Viswanathan, M., Ammerman, A., Eng, E., Garlehner G., Lohr, K. N., Griffith, D., Rhodes, S., Samuel-Hodge, C., Maty, S., Lux, L., Webb, L., Sutton, S. F., Swinson, T., Jackman, A., & Whitener, L. (2004). Community-based partici- patory research: Assessing the evidence. *Evidence Report Technology Assessment (Suppl.)* (99), 1–8.

Wachino, V. (2015). *CMCS Informational Bulletin: Coverage of housing-related activi- ties and services for individuals with disabilities.* Retrieved on June 18, 2021, from https://www.medicaid.gov/federal-policy-guidance/downloads/CIB-06–26 -2015.pdf

Wallerstein, N., & Duran, B. (2017). Theoretical, historical, and practice roots of CBPR. In N. Wallerstein, B. Duran, J. G. Oetzel, & M. Minkler (Eds.). *Community-based participatory research for health: Advancing social and health equity* (3rd ed.) (17–30). Jossey-Bass.

Chapter 5

Substandard Housing in Memphis, Tennessee

*Developing Cross-Sector Collaborations to Address
the Social Determinants of Health*

Christina Plerhoples Stacy, Joseph Schilling, and Steve Barlow

This project illustrates the intersection of housing quality, public health, and strategic code enforcement. Our theory of change reflects the core principles of the social determinants of health—that changes to local government code-enforcement operations and processes for preserving housing quality could set the stage for subsequent improvements in the health of tenants, families, and the community at large.

Reinforcing this work is our team's deep commitment to equity and inclusion in Memphis and beyond. Steve Barlow, the founder and president of Neighborhood Preservation, Inc., has dedicated his life to promoting neighborhood revitalization in Memphis by collaboratively developing practical and sustainable resolutions to blighted properties and to the systems that lead to widespread neglect, vacancy, and abandonment of real estate. Christina Stacy, an economist and senior research associate at the Urban Institute, focuses her work on equity and inclusion in urban spaces, and also spends her free time advocating for and volunteering with affordable housing developers and other equity-focused nonprofits. Joseph Schilling, a former municipal lawyer, facilitator, and senior research associate at the Urban Institute, has spent years working with communities to establish cross-sector collaborations on code enforcement, neighborhood revitalization, and urban regeneration that translates research into policy change on the ground.

In this chapter, we review our work on a strategic policy health impact assessment (HIA) in Memphis, looking at how housing code enforcement could more strategically focus on improving the health and well-being of Memphians. What might seem like a small piece of the puzzle, code enforcement, is really the main line of defense against unhealthy living conditions. And the processes and procedures by which codes are enforced can either improve equity if done properly or reinforce existing inequities if not done in a strategic manner. Our health impact assessment of code enforcement in Memphis produces recommendations for how local code officials can reform their processes and practices and work more closely with its partners (e.g., county health, hospitals, healthcare providers, nonprofits, community organizations, etc.) to improve health equity in the city.

Our team extended the parameters of a traditional health impact assessment from its focus on individual projects or sites to the realm of policy design and development. By using a strategic policy HIA, our project identified and examined a menu of alternative policies, programs, and practices early in the policy process so that local officials, nonprofit partners, and community organizations could assess and develop a holistic and comprehensive approach (e.g., strategic code enforcement) to the health challenges associated with substandard housing in Memphis.

Our research partnership further taught us how important it is to engage community members and practitioners in both the design and implementation of research. Although sometimes quite uncomfortable and challenging, engaging pivotal stakeholders deeply and meaningfully throughout the research process led to a much more useful and impactful outcome.

Where we live matters for our health and well-being. The condition of our homes and neighborhoods can negatively affect our respiratory health (Mudarri & Fisk, 2007; Rauh, Chew, & Garfinkel, 2002; Sharfstein et al., 2001; Shaw, 2004), cognition and neurodevelopment (Bashir, 2002; Coulton et al., 2016; Sharfstein et al., 2001; Shaw, 2004), behavioral health (Bashir, 2002; Burdette, Hill, & Hale, 2011), physical fitness (Bell et al., 2013; Chambers & Rosenbaum, 2013), mental stress (Shonkoff, Boyce, & McEwen, 2009), and physical safety (Cohen et al., 2003; Stacy, 2017).

Homes and apartments with substandard and unhealthy living conditions (e.g., mold, airborne and waterborne lead, malfunctioning appliances, rodents, fire and structural safety hazards, lack of weatherization and utilities, etc.) present communities with serious, complex challenges that demand collaboration among the public, nonprofit, and for-profit sectors to strategically deploy solutions. The first responders to substandard housing, local government code enforcement agencies, typically do not focus on the health impacts of their legal responsibilities to ensure safe and habitable housing within their jurisdictions.[1] Housing code enforcement operations are narrowly structured to administer and enforce applicable state and local housing codes, alleviate structural/safety concerns, and inspect easily visible exterior property conditions rather than protecting and improving the longer-term health of residents. Additionally, code enforcement departments often work in separate local government agencies from public health organizations, making it difficult to

---

1. Throughout this chapter we use the term "code enforcement (CE) agencies" to encompass all local government departments and offices that have compliance and enforcement functions/responsibilities for state and local property, building, health, and environmental codes and regulations; its use is not restricted to those agencies with "code enforcement" in their name. The enforcement function can be housed in different departments within a city or county government, such as housing, neighborhood and community development, zoning, or building inspection.

coordinate and collaborate across sectors (public, private, and nonprofit) to solve substandard housing's interrelated problems.

In Memphis, a city of approximately 652,000 people, a decline in population of 6.4 percent between 2000 and 2010 (U.S. Census Bureau, 2012) and high rates of poverty have contributed to vacant homes in predominately low-income neighborhoods and a housing stock in need of repair. Nearly 40 percent of all occupied housing units in Memphis exhibit at least one of the Census Bureau's physical or financial conditions of poor quality, which include incomplete plumbing or kitchen facilities, more than one occupant per room, and gross rent exceeding 30 percent of a household's income (U.S. Census Bureau, 2016).

The health of Memphis residents is also a concern, with high rates of childhood asthma and chronic diseases concentrated in specific low-income neighborhoods. Childhood asthma affects over ten thousand children in Memphis and was the most common reason for hospitalization in 2015.[2] Among adults, 8.7 percent have asthma, 15.3 percent have diabetes, and 17.8 percent do not have health insurance coverage. Like childhood asthma rates, these health issues are not evenly distributed across the metro region, they are concentrated in lower-income neighborhoods (Memphis Property Hub, n.d.). The County Health Department's work on life expectancy highlights that zip codes with lower life expectancy also have a higher percentage of the population living below the poverty level (Ogari & Sweat, 2016).

What if housing code enforcement agencies could better address these housing and health issues by making public health outcomes a critical policy priority through improved coordination between public

---

2. "Asthma program improves health, lowers healthcare costs," Le Bonheur Children's Hospital, accessed October 13, 2018, http://www.LeBonheur.org/for-providers/physician-publications/delivering-on-a-promise/winter-2014/breathe-easy.dot.

health agencies, community health nonprofits, and the broader system of healthcare institutions?

Our team from the Interdisciplinary Research Leaders (IRL) Program sought to answer that question by conducting a health impact assessment of existing housing code enforcement policies and programs in Memphis, Tennessee (see Stacy et al., 2018a, for the full report and Stacy et al., 2018b, for a short fact sheet summarizing our recommendations). Our core team represented a diverse array of expertise, skills, and interests—Steve Barlow, a practicing lawyer and local leader who started a community development intermediary in Memphis that focuses on property blight elimination; Christina Stacy, an economist with expertise in urban economics and blight; and Joseph Schilling, a nationally recognized expert in municipal law, vacant properties, and code enforcement with a passion for connecting people and creating collaborative learning spaces. We used a blend of qualitative and quantitative data collection and analysis to explore how Memphis housing code enforcement could undertake more strategic and proactive approaches to improve public health outcomes for its neighborhoods with substandard housing.

In this chapter, we define the parameters of our strategic policy health impact assessment and then describe how a community development intermediary[3]—Neighborhood Preservation, Inc. (NPI)—and a research team from the Urban Institute applied the HIA process to create an action plan for local government, hospitals, and community and health

---

3. As an intermediary, NPI performs a wide array of activities within the general sphere of housing and community development, such as convening, policy advocacy, revitalization projects, redevelopment, etc. It acts as a bridge among and between diverse groups of stakeholders and agencies (NPI, n.d.). Within the field, community development financial institutions (CDFIs) represent the more common intermediary, but these roles are expanding to a wider range of entities, as NPI's portfolio illustrates. See generally, MacArthur Foundation, 2016.

nonprofits to address the housing and health problems associated with substandard housing issues in Memphis. As part of the HIA process, we crafted a common policy framework that built a mutual understanding of the health and housing relationships among a wide array of cross-sector stakeholders. With assistance from our community partner, NPI, we brought together local representatives from healthcare, community development, and housing working in city government, county government, the nonprofit sector, and research institutions to identify the ways in which a more strategic approach to housing and neighborhood code enforcement could improve the health and quality of life of residents.

Our community partner, NPI, played multiple roles throughout our project. A fundamental and distinguishing feature of the IRL model is having a community partner involved in the design, execution, and dissemination of the research. Embedding NPI's executive director as part of the team benefited our research greatly because of his ideas, networks, and deep knowledge of community development, housing, and code enforcement in Memphis. NPI was also instrumental in helping us engage with relevant decision-makers and other local stakeholders including experts from the University of Memphis. For example, our team convened a community-based project advisory group consisting of local code enforcement officials, public health practitioners, public housing administrators, community advocates, and local researchers. Two Urban Institute research assistants and three graduate student research assistants from the University of Memphis's schools of public health, law, and urban planning also contributed substantially to the HIA's data collection, analysis, and findings. We applied the underlying IRL philosophy by taking steps throughout the HIA process to include these research assistants in critical project decisions and to seek feedback and buy-in from the community stakeholders.

In summary, our project illustrates: (1) how the HIA process itself can serve as a vehicle for facilitating cross-sector collaboration at the intersection of housing and public health; (2) the pivotal role that intermediaries (in our case NPI) can play in making the collaborative connections critical to put the "culture of health" into practice (e.g., by and among researchers, practitioners, policymakers, sectors, agencies, and disciplines/fields); and (3) that upgrading housing code enforcement operations, while often overlooked, with strategic code enforcement, can become the cornerstone for any community's efforts to reduce the health threats of living in substandard housing.

Health Impact Assessments

When attempting to improve public health and increase health equity, researchers and policymakers often focus on one policy or program at a time. However, the social determinants of health (SDoH) framework suggests a much more complex interrelationship of the built environment and health that demands a portfolio of cross-sector interventions in order to secure significant policy and organizational change. One of the inevitable challenges of focusing on the social and the environmental determinants of health simultaneously is connecting and guiding all the stakeholders and community leaders toward a holistic, coordinated plan of action. Because of the complexities of substandard housing, municipal code enforcement, and public health programs in Memphis, our team adapted the HIA framework to consider a broad range of policy interventions early in the policy and program design stage. In the next section we outline the traditional HIA framework and discuss the design and development of our "strategic policy" HIA.

HIA Overview

HIAs are assessment frameworks that aim to make health a key variable in policymaking. According to Schnake-Mahl and Norman (2017), it is not always clear to elected officials how much of our health is place-based. HIAs allow public health expertise and recommendations to inform decision-making without forcing non–health professionals to digest potentially dense health data (Wernham, 2011). More importantly, they force a discussion of health impacts where they previously may have been overlooked.

Many HIAs have been conducted to assess the potential health impacts of housing, urban planning, and community-development sector policies and programs (Dannenberg et al., 2008). Communities across the country are using this tool to help bridge sectoral divides and explain how implementing proposed policies and strategies will improve the health and well-being of a target population (Suther & Sandel, 2013; Wernham, 2011). In some places, such as Baltimore, Maryland, the results of HIAs are directly influencing the zoning code and land-use planning process for the city (Thornton et al., 2013). Research shows that HIAs have an impact on decision-making processes; one study found that, out of twenty-three HIA studies, fourteen decision-makers reported the associated HIA significantly influenced their decision process (Bourcier et al., 2015).

Traditional HIAs combine stakeholder input with quantitative health data to construct a predictive model based on the potential policy. HIAs consist of six common steps as shown in table 5.1.

Table 5.1   Components of a Health Impact Assessment

Steps	Description
Screen	Identify proposed policy or program within political context
	Analyze feasibility of study, expected resource requirements
	Determine whether HIA would add value to decision-making process
Scope	Identify goals and stakeholders, and develop logic model diagram
	Identify potential health effects
	Identify research questions, data sources, and data gaps
Assess	Undertake literature review, stakeholder analysis
	Undertake data analysis
	Undertake health effects analysis, including baseline analysis
Recommend	Identify proposals and alternatives to mitigate adverse health effects
	Create health management plan
	Identify stakeholders who could implement recommendations
Report	Analyze proposal population affected, stakeholder engagement, data methods, findings, and recommendations
	Communicate recommendations to decision-makers and other stakeholders
Monitor and evaluate	Track changes in implementation of HIA recommendations
	Evaluate if HIA influenced decision-making process

Source: Adapted from National Research Council, 2011.

Our HIA

For our analysis, we modified the traditional HIA framework by looking beyond a single policy, program, or project. Our strategic policy HIA considered a portfolio of policies and programs earlier in the policy design stage so that policymakers, partners, and communities could weigh alternatives and better understand the interrelationship and potential interaction of new with existing policies and programs. For Memphis, our team examined how a more strategic system of housing and health code enforcement (table 5.2) could have a range of health impacts. While

Table 5.2 Steps of the HIA Process

	Screen	Scope	Assess	Recommend	Report	Monitor and evaluate
Goal	Determine whether an HIA is needed	Identify the pathways between code enforcement and potential health impacts	Gather relevant data, assess the pathways between inputs and impacts, and draw conclusions regarding the potential impact of code enforcement	Use the results from the assessment to suggest changes to CE policies and procedures for the benefit of public health	Disseminate findings to decision-makers, affected communities, and the general public	Evaluate the HIA according to accepted standards of practice and monitor and measure its impact on decision-making and health
HIA overview	Identify the program or policy decision(s) that are part of the HIA	Define HIA objectives and goals Refine research parameters	Refine research questions and other important questions	Compile recommendations based on qualitative and quantitative research findings	Work with code enforcement department to create a plan of action based on findings	Work with the code enforcement department and other stakeholders to set up a system to continue to track health outcomes over time
Community engagement	Determine whether and how the HIA will add value for the community through discussions with stakeholders Develop community outreach and engagement plan for the HIA process	Inventory full list of stakeholders Identify and recruit members for advisory committee Convene advisory group Convene first of three community meetings/ focus groups	Convene second meeting of advisory group	Convene second community meeting/ focus group	Convene third community meeting potentially combined with a data walk	Convene third meeting of advisory group

Table 5.2 *(continued)*

	Screen	Scope	Assess	Recommend	Report	Monitor and evaluate
Qualitative research	Develop logic model Conduct preliminary literature review	Design interview guides and interview plan	Conduct interviews and site tours with core Memphis stakeholders Analyze interview data Finalize literature review	Analyze results from qualitative research to synthesize policy recommendations	Use storytelling and other techniques to disseminate qualitative findings (e.g., blog posts)	
Quantitative research	Begin to create inventory of data sources	Finalize data inventory Conduct process mapping for the CE interventions	Collect time series data on CE interventions and health conditions Assess baseline health conditions Map baseline health conditions Describe and map CE interventions Estimate relationship between CE interventions and health outcomes using panel econometric techniques Map final health conditions and overlay with CE interventions	Analyze results from quantitative research to synthesize policy recommendations	Use data visualizations and other quantitative techniques to disseminate quant findings in an accessible way	

a traditional HIA identifies the potential health impacts of a single proposed policy or development project, our strategic policy HIA explored
the health impacts of a current set of policies and practices (all those
related to code enforcement) and identified ways to alter these policies
and practices to more proactively improve public health.

Screen

Bourcier and colleagues (2015) recommend that to maximize the impact
of an HIA, the team should select an issue that is already building social
momentum for change. Therefore, as we began with the screening phase,
in which the HIA team and stakeholders determined whether an HIA
was needed, we consulted with national health policy practitioners, our
Memphis community partner NPI, and a few of their core partners to
learn about the state of local housing and code enforcement efforts in
order to identify relevant issues and related research that would both fill
a gap in the literature and provide an opportunity for change where it
was needed.

   At the time of screening in 2016, the city's housing code enforcement
operation was beginning a transformation, spearheaded by recently
elected Memphis mayor Jim Strickland, who appointed a new director of
the City Code Enforcement Department with substantial code enforcement experience. Additionally, housing and public health stakeholders in
Memphis had recently come together to confront issues related to blight,
code enforcement, and public health. In 2016, leaders from the nonprofit, public, and private sectors collaborated on developing the nation's
first blight elimination charter—a declaration of principles, goals, and
actions that would enable stronger coordination across sectors, agencies,

and community-based organizations working on these issues (Barlow, 2016a, 2016b).

Participants in this strategic planning process convened the first community-wide blight elimination summit in March 2016 to publicly endorse the charter and launch a Blight Elimination Steering Team to propel the charter's recommendations into action. Around the same time, Le Bonheur Children's Hospital and the University of Memphis School of Law convened a broad coalition of local healthcare providers with housing and community development organizations and civic groups to form the Memphis/Shelby County Health Homes Partnership and develop a Green & Healthy Homes Initiative website, which was approved in 2017. Collectively these efforts have enabled local policymakers, practitioners, and researchers to better understand the relationships among health, housing quality, community development, neighborhood revitalization, and crime in Memphis. Given the momentum building toward healthy homes, the timing seemed ideal to explore stronger policy and programmatic connections between healthy housing and code enforcement.

Scope

Once we decided that an HIA was needed and identified the topic area, the team scoped out the work, identifying relationships between code enforcement and potential health impacts. This phase started with a review of the practice literature on code enforcement and research on promising practices from other cities. Our graduate research assistants met with code enforcement officials in Memphis to create maps of the processes they currently use to investigate and inspect properties as well as the different enforcement actions they can take under the current code when they cannot gain voluntary compliance. They finished a similar exercise for the Environmental Court of Shelby County, where Memphis is located. The Environmental Court was created in 1983 by the City of Memphis to handle violations of its health, fire, building, and zoning codes.

Since 2001, the Environmental Court has heard all cases brought under the Abatement of Nuisances Statute. Under this authority, the court has ordered the closing of dozens of crack houses, strip clubs, apartment complexes, and other entities deemed to constitute a public nuisance. Since 2007, the Environmental Court has also heard cases violating the Neighborhood Preservation Act, which addresses substandard vacant buildings that have become public nuisances (Shelby County, Tennessee, n.d.).

In an HIA, community input is crucial to understanding the needs of the populations most directly affected by a potential policy (Heller et al., 2013). Therefore, we convened a project advisory group made up of stakeholders from housing and health nonprofits, public agencies, and community groups to provide input on the research questions and design. This project advisory group would later provide feedback on preliminary findings and final recommendations.

Assess

After scoping out the study and compiling input from local community stakeholders, we turned to assessment, in which we gathered relevant data, undertook a literature review, assessed the pathways connecting inputs and impacts, then drew conclusions about the potential outcomes of possible solutions. This phase involved working with local partners in Memphis to obtain data on all city and county code enforcement practices, along with crime and health data at the smallest possible levels of geography.

Another important dimension of this HIA was the unique ability to blend qualitative engagement with quantitative analysis of relevant data made possible by the development of integrated data systems already initiated in the city. Beginning in early 2015, NPI, together with the Memphis Bloomberg Innovation Team, created the initial version of a real property data portal called the Memphis Property Hub whose primary mission is to document, track, collect, and disseminate existing official local and administrative records concerning each of the real property parcels, especially blighted, vacant, and foreclosed housing that put neighborhoods at risk. The Property Hub acquires all data sets available that include a permanent parcel number or a street address as a searchable identifier and makes it possible to conduct searches of multiple records sources for information associated with those unique real property identifiers. Local members of the Bloomberg Innovations team formed a separate nonprofit, Innovate Memphis, to carry on their work leveraging data as a catalyst for social innovation and policy change. Innovate Memphis now serves as the institutional home for the Property Hub. Through the early versions of this Property Hub, the Memphis HIA team could conveniently access and analyze point-level data on substandard housing, health, and neighborhood characteristics. We analyzed these data, looking for spatial connections and trends among substandard housing, code enforcement, health, and crime.

In addition to quantitative data, we collected and analyzed qualitative interview data from a variety of local Memphis stakeholders in public, private, and nonprofit sectors to identify ways in which code enforcement in Memphis could more strategically target better health as a key outcome. We found stakeholders by conducting an inventory of key actors from relevant city and county agencies involved with substandard housing and vacant properties. This inventory included people from community development corporations, healthcare institutions, public health non-profits, and a sample of private businesses that own and manage rental housing in Memphis. Most of these people were mid-level program and project managers or directors of organizations and initiatives along with some frontline staff.

Based on the stakeholder inventory, our local research team began a series of reconnaissance meetings and focus groups with the core agencies: housing code enforcement, environmental health, the Shelby County Environmental Court (see text box 1), and relevant healthcare institutions and tenant organizations.[4] Our local partner, NPI, was instrumental in helping the team identify, select, recruit, and host many of the meetings and focus groups. During the reconnaissance meetings, the research assistants met with key individuals, typically the mid-level managers and directors of government agencies, and nonprofits involved with housing or health, to understand their roles and programming. Our team then conducted ten focus groups with core stakeholder groups—code enforcement officials, representatives of health and housing nonprofits, landlords, and tenant advocates. The team tailored each interview protocol to capture the particular insights and roles of the different stakeholder groups and to probe deeply their understanding and experiences related to substandard housing as a social determinant of health. Most of the focus groups were done as part of four study visits that engaged one or more of the Urban Institute researchers. Each meeting and focus group uncovered new organizations, stakeholders, and programs that helped

---

4. Given limited resources to undertake interviews of individual tenants and IRB concerns regarding the risks of having tenant focus groups, we were able to capture the plight of tenants living in substandard properties by speaking with the leaders and staff of nonprofit organizations and agencies who work directly with tenants.

us chart the complex landscape of housing and health in Memphis. Our team also developed process maps that chart the processes of the city's housing code enforcement and county Environmental Court to better understand the flow of cases from investigation through enforcement and eventual compliance. These focus groups and supporting qualitative data uncovered a complex landscape of city stakeholders working with these issues and confirmed several policy and programmatic gaps that we found through the quantitative data analysis.

Shelby County Environmental Court

When a code case is litigated, it goes to the Shelby County Environmental Court. This court was established in 1983 to adjudicate issues related to Memphis and Shelby County health, fire, zoning, and building codes (Shelby County, Tennessee, n.d.). Judge Larry Potter, now retired, created the court because he believed that a specialized court could help resolve neighborhood blight and crime issues driven by substandard housing in Memphis and Shelby County (Dries, 2012). The Shelby County Environmental Court began as a city effort to target blight and has transformed into a state-sanctioned county court. The court was the first countywide court in the United States to specifically tackle environmental issues impacting communities. Blighted property remains a significant issue in Memphis and the Environmental Court's statutory powers and tools make it the community's primary venue for resolving issues related to substandard housing and vacant properties when other strategies do not achieve compliance. Based on court data from November 2017, the vast majority of cases are brought to court by the City of Memphis Law Division pursuant to the Tennessee Neighborhood Preservation Act and by the City Code Enforcement Department through administrative citations (author calculations). Of the court cases brought about by the City Code Enforcement Department, 80 percent pertain to single-family properties and 8 percent pertain to multifamily properties (the rest are unknown property types).

Box 1   Shelby County Environmental Court

Next, our research team undertook a stakeholder analysis, which involved organizing the interviews and focus groups into six stakeholder clusters and then assessing stakeholders' respective organizational interests and objectives. This helped us identify common ground, opportunities for cross-agency and cross-sector coordination and collaboration, and potential challenges and barriers to those opportunities. Based on the stakeholder analysis we started to chart the relationships among these critical organizations and institutions to identify potential patterns of alignment or dissonance related to some of the ideas and recommendations for strategic code enforcement policies and practices.

Recommend

Next, we compiled and crowdsourced recommendations for changes to the code enforcement process in Memphis designed to improve the public health outcomes of residents. This phase involved discussions with stakeholders, the project advisory group, and desk research on promising solutions other cities have deployed at the policy and programs intersections of substandard housing and health. It also involved sharing and revising a recommendations document with advisors, key stakeholders, and all team members before settling on a final set of recommendations.

During our analysis of the Memphis data and local code enforcement practices, we were surprised to find that the vast majority of city housing code enforcement service requests only involved conditions outside the home. Memphis housing code enforcement did not seem to have a management process or system for prioritizing community requests based on the severity of the violation and its impact on or threat to public health. Our local project advisory group mentioned a recent outbreak of bedbugs where no city department or county agency was assigned the inspection and enforcement responsibility. Similar gaps in services were found with the inspection, enforcement, and abatement of mold in residential dwellings.

Our maps showed a low correlation between the density of code visits to houses and the number of houses with substandard conditions within a neighborhood, suggesting that code enforcement actions could be better targeted to neighborhoods with housing that experiences greater levels of distress and decline. Additionally, there is little relationship between the prevalence of neighborhood crime and the density of code service requests (and even a negative relationship between property crime and code enforcement), suggesting either that code enforcement is helping to reduce crime (perhaps because reporting of violations is lower in these neighborhoods), or that it is not effectively reaching high-crime neighborhoods. Finally, we found a positive correlation between the density of community requests for code inspections/services and the percentage of houses that are single-family units, suggesting that code enforcement is concentrated in neighborhoods with single-family homes and is not targeting apartments and other multifamily housing (i.e., structures with three or more units) as much as it could be.

Based on these findings, our final HIA Report (Stacy et al., 2018b) recommended that the Memphis City Housing Code Enforcement Department prioritize service requests to focus on violations that have a higher likelihood of causing serious health problems, expand coverage to areas and violations that are currently less covered, make the inspection process more proactive, and increase collaboration among city code, county environmental health, and a number of other health, housing, and financing organizations (see text box 2).

Memphis HIA Final Recommendations

Increase Prioritization

Code enforcement agencies should prioritize violations that are more likely to cause serious health concerns, such as mold (which leads to asthma) and lead (which leads to developmental delays in children).

- Work with public health experts to update policy manuals and prioritization systems to emphasize health-related violations.
- Consider providing code officers with administrative citation authority to impose fines and penalties on routine nonstructural violations like parking on the grass. This would free up time to focus efforts on more serious violations.

Inspect Proactively

Code enforcement agencies should undertake proactive inspections rather than rely solely on the complaint-based system that most code agencies follow.

- Conduct systematic sweeps of problem properties and strategically critical neighborhoods.
- Implement a chronic nuisance ordinance.
- Enhance tenant protections to ensure that these regulatory approaches do not lead to displacement (which may also lead to increased reporting and enhanced coverage).

Broaden Coverage

Code enforcement agencies should expand their coverage to properties currently overlooked by the system and develop a neighborhood typology that will allow for enhanced strategic coverage of the city.

- Fill in gaps in services, such as inspecting for bed bugs and mold.
- Enhance education for residents and code enforcement inspectors about healthy homes and code services.
- Enhance resources for repairs through a housing trust fund, vacant property tax, or other dedicated funding source.

(continued)

Increased Collaboration

Finally, code enforcement agencies and their public, private, and nonprofit partners must develop more opportunities for cross-sector collaboration.
- Improve the referral systems among agencies, health care organizations, and nonprofits.
- Cross train inspectors from different agencies and departments.
- Improve data-sharing systems and use real-time data to prioritize code enforcement and property blight prevention in dwellings and neighborhoods where it is evident that health problems are concentrated.

Box 2   Memphis HIA Final Recommendations

Report

Throughout this process, we disseminated intermediate findings to decision-makers, affected communities, the media, and the general public. This reporting phase intensified in October 2018, when the report was published and presented to local stakeholders at the third annual Blight Summit in Memphis. NPI then took the lead on disseminating the HIA's findings to a variety of different local audiences through presentations at community gatherings and policy-making meetings.

Monitor and Evaluate

Our research team did monitor the initial results and local changes from the HIA work through periodic updates with our community partner NPI and local stakeholders. As part of this process, we met with the project advisory group in March of 2019 (five months after the public release of the HIA) to gather feedback on the usefulness of the HIA thus far, and to brainstorm ways in which its findings could be promoted and implemented. As often seems the case with HIAs, we did not have sufficient time and resources to really monitor local progress or undertake a more in-depth or systematic assessment of the HIA's effects. Meaningful policy changes take time and then it often takes more time before the health and housing impacts become more visible. For those conducting policy-focused HIAs, we would recommend procuring supplemental resources to perform a more complete HIA assessment perhaps one to three years down the road.

Challenges to Our HIA Approach

Two key challenges for our team were our lack of public health expertise and the fact that Urban Institute researchers did not live or work in Memphis. While one member had been a consultant/advisor to an HIA and was a previous Robert Wood Johnson Scholar through its Active Living Research initiative and the other had expertise in housing economics and crime, no one on the team held an advanced degree in public health or had worked for a public health agency.

To engage public health experts in the HIA process, the Memphis team worked with mentors from Johns Hopkins University and the University of Memphis's School of Public Health and hired one of three graduate research assistants from the University of Memphis's School of Public Health. Tapping into university expertise filled the void of public health knowledge. The team's local project advisory group also included several members who were healthcare providers or connected to public health. The project advisory group also helped mitigate the Urban Institute Interdisciplinary research leaders' lack of proximity. Rounding out the NPI project team to provide staff on the ground were two graduate research assistants, one from the University of Memphis Law School who had represented the city before the Shelby County Environmental

Court (a key focus of the HIA) and one from the University of Memphis School of Urban Affairs and Public Policy who had worked with several community development corporations in neighborhoods experiencing the challenges of vacant, blighted properties.

Insights and Lessons for Cross-Sector Collaboration in Health and Housing Policy and Research

Our experience in Memphis highlights the promise of cross-sector collaborations involving city agencies, healthcare providers, academic partners, and other community stakeholders to structure and implement housing, urban planning, and community development policies that consider population health. These collaborations have the potential to transform neighborhoods into healthier places to live. While access to safe, healthy, and affordable housing in stable neighborhoods is an important element of improving population health, we also hope that our effort to apply the IRL model of engaged, community-driven research illustrates the importance of approaching the complexity of the social determinants of health through cross-disciplinary research and teamwork. This can help ensure that local housing code enforcement policies and programs prioritize community needs and underlying health determinants. The HIA process and other tools used here to identify areas for better coordination and cross-disciplinary thinking could be used to resolve gaps in other areas, such as the health implications of policies that affect access to high-quality education, transit, and jobs; and exposure to violence and crime.

In reflecting on the Memphis HIA experience, three essential elements of successful health and housing collaborations emerged: (1) the usefulness of HIAs as a vehicle for cross-sector collaboration; (2) the need for multiple levels and types of translation among policymakers, practitioners, and researchers, and (3) the pivotal role and critical leadership of a highly competent and trusted local intermediary.

HIAs as a Vehicle for Cross-Sector Collaboration

HIAs provide a natural format for cross-sector collaboration, stakeholder engagement, and research translation into concrete policy actions. They serve to bring together stakeholders from multiple disciplines and sectors to consider health while achieving other important policy objectives. Success in optimizing health via housing, urban planning, and community development policy requires a unique set of stakeholders. These include public health, housing, community development, and urban planning professionals. Community representatives, including neighborhood association leaders and informed residents, also need a seat at the table to articulate the ways in which community transformation, housing affordability, and local urban planning policies and programs could affect the quality of their daily lives.

The collaborative nature of an HIA made it the ideal process for bridging the health-housing policy and program service delivery divide in Memphis. NPI's extensive role as convener, facilitator, and community catalyst for neighborhood revitalization ideally positioned it to help lead the outreach and engagement activities for this project. Another important HIA dimension at play with the Memphis project was the ability to blend qualitative analysis with quantitative analysis of relevant data for a more comprehensive perspective on both problems and solutions. On the qualitative front, the research team leveraged the focus groups with the critical housing and health stakeholders who work on or have lived experience with substandard housing and the social determinants of having healthy housing. Through these interviews, the team compiled a more complete inventory of the actors as they identified a range of potential steps that could make substandard housing and code enforcement more strategic. On the quantitative front, beginning in early 2015, NPI, together with the Memphis Bloomberg Innovation Team, created a real property data intermediary called the Memphis Property Hub. Its primary mission was to collect, curate, and disseminate all available public and proprietary data on real property parcels, especial blighted, vacant, and foreclosed homes. With access to this Property Hub, the Memphis HIA team could easily acquire and analyze point-level data on substandard housing, and demographic, health, and neighborhood characteristics for all of Memphis. Using data such as these, as well as census tract-level maps, the team was able to identify where code enforcement was concentrated, where it was lacking (both geographically and in terms of the type of issue addressed), and how it might better address health and health equity by filling in some of these gaps.

Community readiness also contributed to the success of this HIA. Before the HIA, NPI had successfully led several local working groups and initiatives around code enforcement and the elimination of blighted properties, including the 2015 Blight Elimination Charter (Barlow, 2016a). NPI was also involved in the formation of the University of Memphis Law School's neighborhood preservation law clinic (Schaffzin, 2016).[5] Thus, NPI's previous work to raise the visibility of blighted properties and substandard housing, together with the strength of the Environmental Court and the new Property Hub, made the community more open and receptive to engaging in our HIA. As such, we recommend that future HIAs identify a local community-based entity to have as a research partner and include a readiness assessment to the scoping

5. Note that two of our graduate research assistants for the HIA were members of this law clinic.

phase of the HIA to determine whether the community is at the right stage for an HIA.

Multiple Dimensions of Research and Policy Translation

Meaningful collaboration requires those involved to effectively translate each other's unique languages, since different sectors and disciplines often have distinct terminologies and cultures (Hermann, Henry, & Hogan, 2017; Kania & Kramer, 2011). Beyond language, there are translation challenges related to differences in underlying policy priorities and regulatory regimes. For example, in Memphis each division that touches substandard housing and its health impacts often reacts to a different set of policy priorities and regulatory requirements, and sometimes different levels of government. For Memphis, the translation activities seemed to span several critical dimensions and scales, such as mapping the housing and code enforcement processes in Memphis. Process mapping, in these cases, helped public health and housing researchers, policymakers, and practitioners develop a shared understanding of the different policy domains and systems they were all attempting to influence and change. Certainly, these cross-disciplinary activities and discussions were not without challenges. It took considerable energy and focus for each team to create its own cross-disciplinary understanding and effectively design and develop their respective research projects.

Translating health and housing principles, terminology, and practices was a fundamental first step for the community development and health fields, so as to establish a common understanding of complexities and to select interventions that addressed the appropriate policy intersections. For example, the Memphis team's cross-disciplinary group of graduate research assistants allowed us to bring multiple sectors together to discuss overlapping topics while identifying and translating terms that were not commonly used by all parties in the room. One prime example of this is that the abbreviation "CDC" is used to refer to community development corporations by the housing sector, whereas the same abbreviation is used by the public health and health care sectors to reference the Centers for Disease Control and Prevention, a federal agency within the U.S. Department of Health and Human Services. Identifying these differences in terminology and shorthand up front allowed us to minimize miscommunication throughout the process.

Memphis's HIA required in-depth analysis and conversations relating to the diagramming of housing code enforcement processes from inspection through cases filed with the Shelby County Environmental Court. In some ways, the public health researchers and practitioners on the team undertook a crash course in the fundamentals of local government land-use regulation, urban planning, housing code enforcement, and community development. The same could be said in the sphere of public health for the urban planners, economists, and housing and community development leaders. Public health's disciplinary focus on the pathways and drivers of disease, how it varies among populations, and how individual and collective behaviors can increase or decrease the risks of exposure were often new concepts for the community development and urban planning professionals. Building this common understanding was critical for identifying, selecting, and coordinating a cohesive set of public health, housing, and urban planning policies that could effectively address the intersections of health issues across a variety of housing conditions and neighborhood circumstances.

The team focused on the translation of research findings into policies and actions, a key objective of the HIA process. Community action and policy change were embedded into the IRL grant program that required each team to consist of two researchers and one fully engaged community partner. IRL curriculum, group discussions, and virtual workshops focused on concepts and practices of policy change, communications, and outreach. Building on these insights, the team was able to recommend specific policy and program changes on the basis of its comprehensive analysis and conclusions.

A Trusted Local Intermediary

A strong community-based intermediary organization and engaged local public leaders were necessary to facilitate collaboration and translation throughout the HIA process. They will also be critical in building consensus and momentum to implement the recommendations outlined in the final report. As part of our HIA/qualitative analysis we identified several organizations working with multiple entities in various sectors and subject-matter fields on the different dimensions of substandard, vacant, and abandoned property or that provide technical support to those involved in the front lines of Memphis's efforts to restore blighted properties.

NPI and the Memphis Property Hub data portal provide multifaceted support roles within Memphis's ecosystem of organizations seeking to prevent, rehab, and reclaim substandard, vacant, and abandoned properties. NPI administers a number of programs and initiatives that engage all sectors (public, private, and nonprofit) along with its advocacy for policy change in all three sectors. Although the Memphis Property Hub is operated through the University of Memphis Center for Applied Earth Science and Engineering Research (CAESER), its research, analysis, and data curation services support the policies and programs of the other stakeholders, such as the Blight Elimination Steering Team, housing code enforcement, NPI, and other nonprofit and public-sector stakeholders. The Hub and NPI bring additional information capacities and legal expertise that are essential in moving Memphis toward a strategic code enforcement model.

As our IRL community research partner, NPI also played important roles as convener, facilitator, and connector. It is now in effect the steward of our HIA research project and will be responsible for translating the HIA's insights and recommendations into local policy action. Since NPI has strong roots in the community development world in Memphis, the trust it has built through decades of community engagement will enable it to translate the recommendations in a way that is meaningful to local communities and key stakeholders.

Other groups in Memphis also help to coordinate cross-sector collaborations for healthier homes in Memphis, such as the Healthy Homes Partnership, which is a group of Memphis and Shelby County leaders as well as officials from twenty-five partner organizations. The Healthy Homes Partnership has worked with the national Green and Healthy Homes Initiative, a Baltimore-based nonprofit dedicated to producing healthier and more efficient housing, to establish the local Memphis/Shelby County Green and Healthy Homes Initiative site. The Healthy Homes Partnership and local Green and Healthy Homes Initiative program are both led by essentially the same multisector group of health-care providers, public health organizations, housing service providers, legal services entities, and community development organizations. Like NPI, the local Healthy Homes Partnership and the Green and Healthy Homes Initiative participants have an underlying interest in cross-sector collaboration derived from their common goal to improve health through better housing. They also have an immediate interest in building a coalition of health and housing providers who support and follow the Green and Healthy Homes Initiative practice of braiding multiple funding strands to provide comprehensive health and energy-efficiency rehabilitation work to achieve better health outcomes for homeowners and renters.

Green and Healthy Homes Initiative has also been exploring with Le Bonheur Hospital CHAMP (Changing High-Risk Asthma in Memphis through Partnership) and other state and local partners the potential of social innovation funding to support healthy homes services for asthma patients as well as other vulnerable populations, including seniors. The "Pay for Success" model proposes using private sector investments to fund health-focused home rehabilitation and repaying such investment from future cost savings (or value-based payments) by state Medicaid agencies or their managed care organizations.

The University of Memphis School of Public Health, Law School, and School of Urban Affairs and Public Policy also play an interconnecting role. Researchers from each school examine different aspects of health and housing depending on their discipline. A few actually enhance community capacity by engaging graduate students in fieldwork, such as the University of Memphis Cecil B. Humphreys School of Law Neighborhood Preservation Clinic (Barlow, Schaffzin, & Williams, 2017). The university's primary interest is service-learning opportunities and research benefits (e.g., publications, findings). The final group in the intermediary cluster are the local foundations that fund much of the health and housing work, with some recent additional support from national foundations (e.g., Kresge and Robert Wood Johnson Foundations).

In moving the HIA's recommendations into action, it will be critical for NPI and the Healthy Homes Partnership to continue the collaborations they nurtured during our project. In Memphis, as in other communities, housing and health organizations and their individual leaders in the public service, public interest, and private sectors are starting to know each other and enhancing their understanding of how housing conditions and neighborhood environments determine the health of residents. Healthy Homes Partnership seems to provide a forum for maintaining these individual and organizational connections and relationships in Memphis. However, this is a relatively new phenomenon and a critical first step in laying the groundwork for collective action. The role of NPI and Healthy Homes Partnership in leadership and coordination will be critical in maintaining momentum toward healthier housing and neighborhoods going forward.

Conclusion and Next Steps

There are numerous opportunities for building on the Memphis example. This study uncovered the complexities that arise in coordinating across community development, neighborhood revitalization, housing, and health. Cross-site research that compares different approaches across different cities to identify common elements and unique community characteristics could help establish closer connections between health and neighborhood revitalization programs and policies. Furthermore, while HIAs are a key mechanism for incorporating health perspectives into non-health-subject policymaking, it is still necessary to move beyond HIA to policy assessment and program evaluation following adoption of more collaborative and coordinated interventions. This evaluation of impacts should be cross-sector and interdisciplinary as well but still in keeping with the stated goals/priorities of a given policy.

From a public health perspective, the insights and lessons from Memphis about better coordination across each of the varying social determinants of health and healthcare institutions would help to not only lessen illness and alleviate health issues, but also prevent them in the first place. And a greater focus on prevention of illness could save money by eliminating the root causes of health inequities rather than merely treating symptoms with Band-aids, inhalers, and emergency room visits. As a first step, our strategic HIA served as a diagnostic tool to identify relevant and promising policy and programmatic pathways that could improve health outcomes for tenants and adjacent residents. The HIA did support several programmatic reforms, such as expanding the partnership with the local Green and Healthy Homes Coalition, elevating the cross-agency environmental health inspection team, and the drafting of a citywide rental inspection ordinance. We hope these initial reforms will serve as the building blocks for more robust policy initiatives around substandard housing and health that can support more meaningful systems change that will be necessary to address the deeper roots of structural racism that perpetuate health and housing disparities.

Improving neighborhoods and population health takes a concerted effort across multiple policy dimensions as well as ongoing coordination among multiple sectors with competing demands and priorities to ensure that there are neither duplication nor gaps in practice and service delivery programs. Lessons learned from the Memphis Strategic Code Enforcement HIA lend insight into how sectors can work together to address the upstream social and environmental determinants of health.

References

Barlow, S. (2016a, March 17). *Memphis neighborhood blight elimination charter.* Retrieved June 4, 2021, from http://www.memphisfightsblight.com/wp-content/uploads/2016/12/Blight_Elimination_Charter_final_3–14-15.pdf

Barlow, S. (2016b, December 13). *Memphis fights blight: Collaborating to win the battle against vacant and abandoned property.* Federal Reserve Bank of St. Louis.

Retrieved June 4, 2021, from https://www.stlouisfed.org/publications/bridges/fall-2016/memphis-fights-blight

Barlow, S. E., Schaffzin, D. M., & Williams, B. J. (2017). Ten years of fighting blighted property in Memphis: How innovative litigation inspired systems change and a local culture of collaboration to resolve vacant and abandoned properties. *Journal of Affordable Housing and Community Development Law, 25*(3), 347–389. Retrieved March 30, 2021, from http://www.jstor.org/stable/26427340.

Bashir, S. A. (2002). Home is where the harm is: Inadequate housing as a public health crisis. *American Journal of Public Health, 92*(5), 733–738.

Bell, J., Mora, G., Hagan, E., Rubin, V., & Karpyn, A. (2013). Access to healthy food and why it matters: A review of the research. PolicyLink.

Bourcier, E., Charbonneau, D., Cahill, C., & Dannenberg, A. L. (2015). An evaluation of health impact assessments in the United States, 2011–2014. *Preventing Chronic Diseases, 12,* 140476.

Burdette, A. M., Hill, T. D., & Hale, L. (2011). Household disrepair and the mental health of low-income urban women. *Journal of Urban Health: Bulletin of the New York Academy of Medicine, 88*(1), 142–153.

Chambers, E. C., & Rosenbaum, E. (2013). Cardiovascular health outcomes of Latinos in the affordable housing as an Obesity Mediating Environment (AHOME) study: A study of rental assistance use. *Journal of Urban Health: Bulletin of the New York Academy of Medicine, 91*(3), 489–498.

Cohen, D. A., Mason, K., Bedimo, A., Scribner, R., Basok, V., & and Farley, T. A. (2003). Neighborhood physical conditions and health. *American Journal of Public Health, 93*(3), 467–471.

Coulton, C., Fischer, R. L., Richter, F. G.-C., Kim, S.-J., & Cho, Y. (2016). Housing crisis leaves lasting imprint on children in Cleveland. MacArthur Foundation.

Dannenberg, A. L., Bhatia, R., Cole, B. L., Heaton, S. K., Feldman, J. D., & Rutt, C. D. (2008). Use of health impact assessment in the U.S.: 27 case studies 1999–2007. *American Journal of Preventative Medicine, 34*(3), 241–256.

Dries, Bill. (2012, January 27). Potter reflects on 30-year tenure as Environmental Court judge. *Memphis Daily News.* Retrieved June 4, 2021, from https://www.memphisdailynews.com/news/2012/jan/27/potter-reflects-on-30-year-tenure-as-environmental-court-judge/print

Heller, J., Malekafzali, S., Todman, L. C., & Wier, M. (2013). Promoting equity through the practice of health impact assessment. PolicyLink.

Herrmann, L. C., Henry, B., & Hogan, L. (2017). Building collective impact to improve health and reduce obesity among children: A report on a participatory research approach. *American Journal of Health Studies, 32*(2), 111–136.

Innovate Memphis. (n.d.). What we do. Retrieved June 4, 2021, from https://innovatememphis.com/about/

Kania, J., & Kramer, M. (2011). Collective impact. *Stanford Social Innovations Review, 9*(1), 36–41.

Krieger, J. W., Song, L., Takaro, T. K., & Stout, J. (2000). Asthma and the home environment of low-income urban children: Preliminary findings from the Seattle–King County Healthy Homes Project. *Journal of Urban Health, 77* (1): 50–67.

MacArthur Foundation. (2016, August 4). Using intermediaries for impact. Retrieved June 4, 2012, from https://www.macfound.org/press/article/using-intermediaries-impact

Memphis Property Hub. (n.d.).Reports on Memphis demographics. Retrieved October 13, 2018, from https://memphisfightsblight.policymap.com/maps

Mudarri, D., and Fisk, W. J. (2007). Public health and economic impact of dampness and mold. *Indoor Air, 17*(4), 334.

National Research Council. (2011). *Improving health in the United States: The role of health impact assessment.* National Academies Press.

Neighborhood Preservation, Inc. (NPI). (n.d.). Revitalizing Memphis neighborhoods one property at a time. Retrieved June 4, 2021, from https://npimemphis.org/

Ogari, L., & Sweat, D. (2016). *Seeing is believing: Patterns of life expectancy, poverty, equity and health in Shelby County, TN.* Shelby County Health Department, Office of Epidemiology.

Rauh, V. A., Chew, G. R., & Garfinkel, R. S. (2002). Deteriorated housing contributes to high cockroach allergen levels in inner-city households. *Environmental Health Perspectives, 110* (Suppl. 2), 323–327.

Schaffzin, D. M. (2016). (B)light at the end of the tunnel? How a city's need to fight vacant and abandoned properties gave rise to a law school clinic like no other. *Washington University Journal of Law and Policy, 52*(1), 115. https://openscholarship.wustl.edu/law_journal_law_policy/vol52/iss1/12

Schnake-Mahl, A., & Norman, S. (2017). *Building healthy places: How are community development organizations contributing?* Joint Center for Housing Studies of Harvard University.

Sharfstein, J., Sandel, M., Kahn, R., & Bauchner, H. (2001). Is child health at risk while families wait for housing vouchers? *American Journal of Public Health, 91*(8), 1191–1193.

Shaw, M. (2004). Housing and public health. *Annual Review of Public Health, 25,* 397–418.

Shelby County, Tennessee. (n.d.). History of Environmental Court. Retrieved June 4, 2021, from https://www.shelbycountytn.gov/2125/History-of-Environmental -Court

Shonkoff, J. P., Boyce, W. T., & McEwen, B. S. (2009). Neuroscience, molecular biology, and the childhood roots of health disparities: Building a new framework for health promotion and disease prevention. *Journal of the American Medical Association, 301,* 2252–2259.

Stacy, C. P. (2017). The effect of vacant building demolitions in crime under depopulation. *Journal of Regional Science, 58* (1), 100–115.

Stacy, C. P., Schilling, J., Barlow, S., Gourevitch, R., Meixell, B., Modert, S., Crutchfield, C., Sykes-Wood, E., & Urban, R. (2018a). *Strategic housing code enforcement and public health.* Urban Institute.

Stacy, C. P., Schilling, J., Barlow, S., Gourevitch, R., Meixell, B., Modert, S., Crutchfield, C., Sykes-Wood, E., & Urban, R. (2018b). *Recommendations for strengthening code enforcement for public health.* Urban Institute.

Suther, E., & M. Sandel. (2013). Health impact assessments. *Rhode Island Medical Journal, 96*(13), 27–30.

Thornton, R.L.J., Greiner Safi, A., Fichtenberg, C. M., Feingold, B. J., Ellen, J. M., & Jennings, J. (2013). Achieving a healthy zoning policy in Baltimore: Results of a health impact assessment of the TransForm Baltimore zoning code rewrite. *Public Health Reports, 128*(Suppl. 3), 87–103.

U.S. Census Bureau. (2012, December). Summary population and housing characteristics: 2010. Retrieved June 4, 2021, from https://www.census.gov/library/ publications/2012/dec/cph-1.html

U.S. Census Bureau. (2016). *American Community Survey,* table DP04. Retrieved June 4, 2012, from https://data.census.gov/cedsci/table?g=0400000US47_1600000U S4748000&d=ACS%205-Year%20Estimates%20Data%20Profiles&tid=ACS DP5Y2016.DP04

Wernham, A. (2011). Health impact assessments are needed in decision making about environmental and land-use policy. *Health Affairs, 30*(5), 947–956.

Chapter 6

Exercising Opportunities to Improve the Health of Public Housing Residents through a Housing Authority and Nursing School Partnership

Donna J. Biederman, Ann Michelle Hartman, Irene C. Felsman, Heather Mountz, Tammy Jacobs, Natalie Rich, Laura Fish, and Devon Noonan

The well-established community-campus partnership between the Durham Housing Authority (DHA) and the Duke University School of Nursing (DUSON) described in this chapter is rooted in both entities' desire to improve the health of and decrease health disparities for Durham's public housing residents. DUSON's faculty, staff, and students understand very well that housing is a social contributor to health, and the school's mission encompasses improving the quality of life for members of our local and global society. DUSON students exercise this commitment through health promotion activities in DHA's public housing communities and, when needs dictate, other related interventions. Over time, our partnership has expanded to include several community-based participatory research projects.

Our collaborative work is a direct response to community-identified needs. DHA welcomes the diverse resources available at DUSON including student, staff, and faculty time and expertise as we strive to improve the lives of public housing residents and, in turn, make Durham a healthier and happier place to live. DUSON students, faculty, and staff benefit from the opportunity for applied work in the community with tangible results.

Although both DHA and DUSON are committed to resident health and health improvement, there are challenges in maintaining a strong partnership. Honest, open relationships and respectful communication are key to successful programs, interventions, and research efforts. It is imperative to remember that the ultimate goal of partnerships is to benefit the health of individuals and families in the community.

Contributors to this chapter include Tammy Jacobs (DHA), Natalie Rich (Durham County Department of Public Health), Donna Biederman, Ann Michelle Hartman, Irene C. Felsman, Heather Mountz, and Devon Noonan (DUSON), and Laura Fish (Duke Cancer Institute).

The connection between health and housing is well established. Persons who are precariously housed have worse health outcomes than those who live in more stable circumstances (Aidala et al., 2016; Baker et al., 2017; Singh et al., 2019). In addition, persons living in public housing have diminished health compared to privately housed individuals (Ruel et al., 2010). Public housing authorities and public housing residents stand to benefit from authentic relationships with academic partners through engagement with faculty and students on health-related topics, opportunities for grant funding, and community-based participatory research. Academicians and students could benefit from the experience of partnership with housing authorities and public housing residents to better understand the intricacies of providing housing and how housing affects life experiences, including health. This chapter describes the well-established relationship between the Duke University School of Nursing and the Durham Housing Authority. The evolution of the relationship, our work in improving the health of DHA residents while advancing nursing education and science, and the benefits and challenges of our partnership are explored.

Background
Public Housing and Health

Housing is an essential social contributor to health. Housing not only provides safety from the elements, but also offers a sense of identity, a place for socialization, and a space to live life as one sees fit. These experiences are related to the overall quality of the housing and neighborhood dynamics. In general, persons with higher socioeconomic positions live in higher-quality housing with neighborhood dynamics that support healthier opportunities to live, grow, and age.

Public housing was instituted in the United States during the Great Depression as part of Franklin Delano Roosevelt's New Deal. Many New Deal, and later Great Society, programs were intended to improve the overall living conditions of impoverished families, the disabled, and older adults. Currently, public housing is varied in design (e.g., single-family dwellings, duplexes, high-rise apartments) and is administered by local housing authorities through funding from the U.S. Department of Housing and Urban Development (HUD). Research has demonstrated that people living in public housing have worse health than those in other housing situations (Ruel et al., 2010) and engage in less healthy behaviors (Noonan et al., 2017).

Durham Housing Authority

DHA was established in 1949 to address substandard housing issues for impoverished persons in Durham, North Carolina. At that time, the population of the city of Durham was reported as 70,307 (U.S. Department of Commerce, Bureau of the Census, 1950). By the mid-1950s two housing projects, the first for White residents and the second for Black residents, were constructed, offering the city's initial 487 units of public housing to low-income families (DHA, 2021). Over the past seventy years, Durham has had substantial population growth and, in 2018, had an estimated 316,739 residents (U.S. Census Bureau, 2020). In turn, the number of units of DHA public housing has increased. As of January 2020, DHA administers twelve public housing properties in Durham, comprising 1,409 units. These sites include properties specifically for families and for elderly or disabled adults within single-story duplexes, two-story apartment complexes, and high-rise buildings. Each property has a resident-elected Resident Advisory Committee that advocates for residents and serves as a liaison between the residents and the DHA administration. Residents benefit from having a Resident Opportunities and Self-Sufficiency Service (ROSS) coordinator who acts as a conduit between the housing authority and community resources. The properties are no longer racially segregated; however, the majority of DHA residents are persons of color.

Community and Nursing School Partnership to Affect Community Health Improvement

Community-campus partnerships can be advantageous to academic partners and their students as well as staff and residents who live and work in public housing. Nursing students and faculty can work with housing authorities on a multitude of projects including community assets and needs identification and collaborative program planning, implementation, and evaluation. Interventions may include health screening and monitoring, health education and coaching, and psychosocial support. Public housing locations offer a rich learning environment for nursing students to understand housing and its impacts on, and relationship with, health outcomes. Such environments allow students to apply the nursing practice model (i.e., the nursing process of assess, diagnose, plan, implement, and evaluate), explore principles of public health, and gain a deeper understanding of the drivers of health. Importantly, in addition to benefitting nursing students, these activities can be a direct benefit to public housing residents who may be underutilizing the healthcare system due to mistrust, financial reasons, or other barriers.

The Duke University School of Nursing Accelerated Bachelor of Science in Nursing (ABSN) program is a second degree program that prepares students with a previous undergraduate degree for practice as professional registered nurses. The DUSON ABSN program was established in 2002 as a response to the growing nursing shortage and has graduated almost 1,700 students since that time. As per the American Association of Colleges of Nursing (AACN) guidelines, the program focuses on health, wellness, and disease prevention as well as evidence-based nursing practice and culturally relevant care (AACN, 2008). In their second semester, DUSON ABSN students complete a portion of their clinical hours in a community-based setting where health outcomes of individuals and populations may be poorer due to poverty, immigration status, or age. Students work in groups of six to eight with a clinical instructor (CI) who is a registered nurse with a minimum of a bachelor of science in nursing degree and at least two years of clinical nursing experience. Because of longstanding professional partnerships, a number of these clinical experiences have taken place in collaboration with organizations that address housing needs in Durham.

In 2011, DUSON and DHA entered into a formal partnership by signing a clinical affiliation agreement that established DHA as an official DUSON ABSN community health clinical site. These types of agreements are essential to allow health professions students the opportunity to learn in real-world settings. The nursing school considered and approached DHA due to the unmet medical needs, lack of access to care, and the diversity of DHA residents across the lifespan. DHA administration was quick to realize the potential positive outcomes of having nursing students and faculty engaged with residents at their properties. The first group of DUSON ABSN students worked with DHA family residents at a summer camp for children. In 2012, a DHA resident from JJ Henderson Towers, a housing site for elderly or disabled adults, approached a DUSON ABSN clinical group and CI at another community clinical site and inquired why they were not involved with the older adult and disabled population at DHA specifically. This resident initiated an introduction to the ROSS coordinator and an invitation to visit the property; this was the catalyst for the long-term relationship that our two organizations enjoy today. Since 2011, DUSON and DHA have had a continuous affiliation agreement that supports DUSON faculty, student, and staff involvement with DHA residents who live in a variety of DHA properties. Funds to support the work that DUSON students do with these communities comes from the ABSN program's operating budget as well as a series of foundation grants.

Evolution of DUSON/DHA Relationship

DUSON Student and Faculty Engagement with DHA Residents

Over the years, the relationship between DUSON and DHA has matured. While DUSON's position has always been to respond to community-identified needs, there is now a clear process to facilitate resident involvement. Students, with the guidance of their CI, conduct a community assets and needs assessment that includes windshield/walking surveys to better understand the surrounding community, and key participant interviews with DHA residents, informal and formal community leaders, and staff to better understand current health priorities. Data generated are then refined through focus groups with DHA residents to clarify the answers to any questions and aid in setting the partnership agenda for the given semester. Students then formulate a ten-week intervention plan with clear objectives. Students implement the plan in weekly three-to-four-hour session with residents; each session culminates in a debriefing session led by the CI. It is through this process that nursing students operationalize the nursing process within a community setting. At the end of the semester, students formally present their project with their peers, faculty, CIs, and community partners in attendance. Generally two to three community representatives from each partner agency are in attendance for the presentation and participate in the post-presentation discussion.

Intervention activities are focused primarily on health screening and referral (e.g., blood pressure for hypertension, body mass index for overweight or obesity, blood glucose or hemoglobin A-1C for diabetes screening), health education, and related wellness and health promotion activities unless other needs are presented by the community as needing attention. In one instance, residents in a family housing development expressed concern about being unprepared to respond to the needs of their families and neighbors in times of crisis and asked for help in gaining skills in communication and in identifying resources for referral purposes. This group of residents participated in a tailored Community Health Advocate course that culminated in a formal ceremony held at

DUSON where the residents wore graduation regalia. This was a very meaningful experience for these residents and many invited their families to attend the graduation ceremony and reception. On another occasion, residents expressed safety concerns due to the level of gang activity at the basketball court and in the playground at the DHA property where they resided. This group participated in a "Take Back Our Park" initiative, which began with a park cleanup event attended by residents, DUSON students and their CI, Durham city police, and the Durham County Sherriff's office. After the cleanup, the students hosted group activities in the park weekly during the semester and assisted residents in writing a grant proposal to a local funder for new playground equipment. The grant was not awarded, but the grant identification and writing process increased resident council members' capacity for similar work in the future. Further, at the request of residents, police increased patrols in the area. The residents expressed that they felt safer at the park and planned to use it on a regular basis.

Over time, we found new ways to engage DHA residents in DUSON ABSN classes beyond community health. For instance, DHA elderly residents came to the DUSON geriatric clinical preparation day to teach students how to appropriately engage with elders on topics of health and healthcare. DHA residents have also served as standardized patients, a paid position, for nurse practitioner students. The residents are routinely reminded that they are truly teaching DUSON students and gratitude is expressed through end-of-semester recognition events.

Because of the responsiveness of the DUSON team and the success of their efforts, a trusting relationship between DUSON and DHA has evolved, which affords the opportunity for more sophisticated projects. These include several unfunded research projects. One such project was a survey that DHA administrative staff developed to better understand why resident attendance at non-mandatory events was low. Following Duke Health's institutional review board (IRB) approval, students and their CI administered the survey, analyzed the data, and presented the deidentified aggregated findings to DHA residents and administration. Another research project was a survey to estimate the prevalence of Adverse Childhood Experiences (ACEs) in adults living at DHA and measure individual resilience. Due to the potential to evoke past trauma from administration of the ACEs and resilience surveys, a group comprising DUSON faculty, CIs, and students; DHA administrators and residents; other faculty at Duke with ACEs experience; and representatives from the local behavioral health managed care organization (MCO) met multiple times to discuss the best approach to gathering these types of data. Surveys were administered to a convenience sample of residents who attended six health fairs within their community. Students administered the survey with residents in a private place with a behavioral health specialist from the MCO immediately available in case the resident needed (or desired) emergent mental health attention. This study, too, received IRB approval and DHA received aggregated deidentified results.

DUSON and DHA Community-Engaged Research

Catalyzed by observations made during nursing clinical site collaborations with DHA, DUSON faculty approached the ROSS coordinator about doing a research study. The study, funded by the DUSON Center for Nursing Research and conducted to inform programming at DHA property sites, sought to determine the prevalence of modifiable health behaviors, including smoking, alcohol use, physical activity, and fruit and vegetable intake among DHA residents, and the corresponding barriers to and facilitators of engaging in healthy behaviors in public housing. Our prior relationship with the ROSS coordinator was key to the success of this project. Since the ROSS coordinator's role is to ensure that elderly and disabled residents continue to live independently in the public housing, we chose to focus the assessment on properties that collectively housed the majority of elderly and disabled residents. The ROSS coordinator was involved in the study from conception through publication including: (1) Assisting with selecting measures to include and the best modality to deploy the survey; (2) community recruitment; (3) providing transportation for some residents to attend focus groups at DUSON; and (4) disseminating results back to the community. Results of the study indicated that residents scored worse than population norms on most health behaviors (Noonan et al., 2017). Rates of smoking were very high and almost double that of population norms (CDC, 2019).

Because of these high smoking rates and a U.S. Department of Housing and Urban Development mandate that all public housing units become smoke-free by August 2018 (HUD, 2016), we anticipated a need for more accessible smoking cessation services. DUSON and Duke faculty researchers worked with DHA staff and the local health department to increase access to smoking cessation support at DHA. This effort started by attending a Resident Advisory Council comprising Resident Advisory Committee chairs from each of the twelve DHA properties and conducting a listening session around the new HUD mandate. We asked what smoking-related services would be beneficial to residents. Results of the listening session indicated that the residents wanted more access to free Nicotine Replacement Therapy (NRT) and readily available programing onsite to assist with quitting. Therefore, building on our prior collaborations, DUSON faculty researchers worked with DHA and the Durham County Department of Health tobacco education specialist to develop a sustainable community health advisor (CHA) tobacco cessation program that could be implemented in DHA communities.

We sought to create a team of DHA residents who were natural helpers in the community and who were eager to support smoking cessation among residents to serve as CHAs and deliver cessation interventions in DHA properties, as well as to co-develop and pilot test the program. To recruit residents to be CHAs, DHA colleagues were asked to recommend individuals based on their knowledge of the communities. Flyers were posted at housing sites and recruitment took place at community events. Potentially eligible DHA residents were invited to complete a standard application form. The application form included questions about smoking history, DHA residency history, prior community involvement, and ideas for improving the health of the DHA community. Five CHA candidates with personal tobacco use experience, and who demonstrated commitment to improving the health of area residents, were hired. Building capacity of community partners is essential to developing a sustainable, community-based program (Goytia et al., 2013) and therefore the CHAs were offered training in fundamentals of research, the American Lung Cancer Association Cessation Navigator training, training in motivational interviewing, and education about local cessation resources to link residents to services.

The CHAs, DHA staff, and researchers worked together to develop the Fresh Life Program, which involved weekly CHA-run office hours for cessation counseling, distribution of NRT to those attempting cessation, and community smoking-cessation events and classes. DHA residents on the team were paid $15 per hour for their time, which included biweekly two-hour team meetings, weekly office hours at their properties, attending or facilitating community events related to promoting smoking cessation at DHA, and any time spent meeting with residents advising about smoking cessation. The CHAs have been providing services under the Fresh Life Program to residents for the past year and results of the program are currently being evaluated.

As this study was progressing, another funded study partnership between DUSON and DHA was also under way. In 2016, the Duke Clinical and Translational Science Institute (CTSI) began a community road-mapping process to identify high-priority community health needs. A series of well-attended community-focused town hall–type meetings ensued where fifty-one unique health related issues were identified. These issues were rank ordered: mental health, heart disease, education, access to affordable housing, cancer, diabetes, and obesity claimed top priority. A workgroup was developed for each of these seven priority areas. Each workgroup facilitated meetings over an eight-month period to develop research questions that could be used for a population health grant through the CTSI. The housing workgroup was routinely attended by representatives from DHA, DUSON, the Durham City Development Office, community-based nonprofit agencies, and community residents. This group decided to explore the mental and physical health correlates of eviction from public housing. A DUSON faculty member and the DHA director of strategic management wrote a grant to the CTSI that was funded for $25,000 for a one-year period. The two were co–principal investigators (PIs) on the study, which necessitated DHA providing information on the number of residents evicted during a five-year period. DHA and Duke University developed data-sharing agreements to allow for data transfer. We discovered that DHA evictions data were not readily available in an electronic format from all its public housing sites. The team worked together to develop a novel mechanism to identify persons who were likely to have been evicted based on individual property financial records (Biederman et al., in press). As of this writing, the study is completed, the PIs have co-presented it twice, an article from the study was published, and another is under review. Study results indicated an increase in five of ten diagnostic categories and increased hospital and emergency department utilization post eviction (Biederman et al., in review), but fewer missed primary care appointments (Callejo-Black et al., 2021).

Prior to the study, DHA was working with the local mental health provider to decrease evictions through financial literacy classes: failure to pay rent is the reason most people are evicted. Understanding the medical diagnoses of persons evicted may inform this and future interventions. Patterns discovered in the financial data, such as the same person incurring multiple notices and fees for late rent payments over time, have already resulted in interventions to alert property managers to identify these residents earlier in the multistage eviction process. Throughout the study period, DHA staff were engaged partners who were sincerely working to better understand the medical vulnerabilities of their residents. During one presentation, an audience member asked why DHA would be so transparent as to publicly acknowledge the number of residents it had evicted. Interestingly, the number was much lower than commonly speculated among community members and increased DHA's credibility as a responsive landlord.

Opportunities for Continued and Enhanced Engagement

In 2016, DUSON adopted a five-year strategic plan that included community health as one of the five priority focus areas. This was the first time in its history that community health was included as a strategic priority at the school. DUSON faculty members who were working with community-based organizations convened and developed goals and strategies to improve community health through partnership, research, education, and programs. As a result, the DUSON Community Health Improvement Partnership Program (D-CHIPP) director Donna

Biederman, who is a coauthor on this book chapter and co-PI on a previously mentioned research study with DHA, was appointed July 1, 2017, and D-CHIPP was launched. The D-CHIPP director works with Heather Mountz, the program coordinator, advisory board, and faculty, staff, and student affiliates. D-CHIPP serves as a bridge between DUSON and the Durham community in efforts to improve community health through research, education, clinical practice, and service.

Recently D-CHIPP received a competitive Intellectual Community Planning Grant through the Duke Provost's Office. The proposal had a specific focus on health equity with housing as a target area for improvement. With these monies, D-CHIPP will engage a multidisciplinary group of researchers from the Duke Schools of Nursing and Medicine, the Duke Sanford School of Public Policy, the Duke Nicholas School of the Environment, and North Carolina Central University with DHA leadership and residents to set a much larger research agenda. The ICPG will allow us to explore community health concerns relating to social, economic, and environmental factors most important to our partners. This will be achieved through a series of meetings and a workshop, with the goal of identifying key issues for which interventions may be designed to positively influence community health outcomes.

Overcoming Obstacles

The DUSON-DHA partnership has been productive for both parties, but it has not been without difficulties. Over the years we have met with various obstacles from both the nursing education and research perspectives. Developing community-campus partnerships that support the learning needs of nursing students can pose several challenges (Thompson & Buchner, 2013). Nursing students must be supervised by a registered nurse and usually work in groups of six to ten students. Public housing authorities do not typically employ registered nurses, so a CI is necessary to oversee the work of the students or another arrangement for distance-based supervision negotiated. Also, students are more accustomed to traditional acute care clinical placements such as in clinic or hospital settings and may need more support, guidance, and time to implement community-based interventions (Bavenko-Mould, Ferguson, & Atthill, 2016) such as the work described above at DHA. A focused community health clinical preparation day, which includes time to explore their community partner organizations and scenarios developed from interactions with DHA residents, has helped students understand the need for and importance of this type of clinical rotation. This is complimented by the overarching DUSON ABSN curriculum that includes implicit bias awareness, cultural intelligence training, and a focus on structural racism.

Public housing sites must also be capable of supporting groups of students that change each semester or even go an entire semester with no student engagement. Time is a limiting factor for building strong community-campus partnerships (Mayer, Braband, & Killen, 2017).

During the initial years of our relationship building, DUSON faculty and staff frequented DHA properties and attended community events between and during off semesters. Thus, the DUSON faculty and staff members maintained the relationship over time to establish a true bilateral partnership rather than giving the appearance that DHA is a convenience for DUSON students. The relationship with the DHA ROSS coordinator and other DHA administrators is strengthened through quarterly networking meetings hosted by DHA. Approximately thirty people representing various organizations in Durham attend these meetings, always including one or two representatives from DUSON and

D-CHIPP. Also, D-CHIPP hosts a small quarterly breakfast meeting with faculty, staff, the DHA ROSS coordinator, and another DHA administrator. These gatherings allow time for fellowship on a personal level to further strengthen the partnership.

Several things were learned through partnering with DHA staff and residents on research. Although the ROSS coordinator was instrumental in publicizing and in recruiting residents to the first collaborative study to understand health behaviors, even with DHA staff support engagement with residents remained difficult. This challenge informed the use of residents to help develop and deliver interventions for a second study on modifiable health behaviors, specific to smoking cessation. Lessons were gleaned about recruiting, hiring, and retaining CHAs to provide smoking cessation services. These include:

- Given the connections that CHAs have in the community, it may be beneficial to consider expanding the focus of the CHAs' work beyond smoking cessation to include other health behaviors, stress and mental health, and other similar smoking-related chronic disease prevention and management activities.
- Word-of-mouth recruitment of CHAs from DHA staff and recruitment at community-based events had the best potential to find the true natural helpers in the DHA community.
- Conducting verbal, in-person applications for the CHA position with simple questions was the best way to reach a diverse pool of applicants and candidates—not everyone has internet or computer access or experience working with computers.
- Communication with CHAs was most acceptable via phone or text.
- To retain CHAs, keeping meetings consistent—same time, same day of the week, same place—convenient, and child-friendly was beneficial.

- Providing food at meetings was preferable.
- Providing training for CHAs that expanded their knowledge base was important to build capacity and keep residents interested and engaged in the program.

Correspondingly, the study supported the work objectives of the ROSS coordinator, including improving resident self-sufficiency through being employed and earning income as a CHA.

Ongoing challenges our team has faced include payment of our CHAs. Initially, we planned to pay CHAs $15 per hour for eight hours a month. As the Fresh Life project gained momentum, several CHAs worked more than that and earning this extra income negatively impacted their income-based benefits (e.g., rent, SSI, Medicaid). We are working with DHA to ensure that CHAs do not have to pay higher rent as a result of income earned doing CHA work. Further, we are working individually with CHAs to link them to advocacy resources for their specific situations. It may not be optimal to prioritize smoking over more pressing issues. We learned to be flexible with agendas and events and sensitive to the needs of the community. For example, when there is community violence or trauma, we take time during meetings to process and grieve or even cancel events to allow residents to process trauma.

Conclusions

A strong community-academic partnership between a city housing authority and a nursing school has the potential to contribute to improving resident health and wellbeing while enhancing nursing student education and community-based participatory research. The examples of community-engaged programs, interventions, and research presented here illustrate the benefits of partnerships between a nursing school and a community public housing organization. However, such a partnership requires a substantial commitment of time from both parties in terms of long-term planning, implementation of programming, and evaluation of outcomes. Honest, open relationships and respectful communication are key to successful programs, interventions, and research efforts. It is imperative to recognize that the ultimate goal of partnerships is to benefit the health of individuals and families in the community.

Acknowledgments

We would like to acknowledge and thank the DHA residents who routinely contribute to the education of DUSON's nursing students through attending clinical programming events and the Fresh Life CHAs for the time and expertise they contributed to improving the health and lives of their neighbors.

A portion of this chapter appeared in Biederman D.J., Hartman A.M., Felsman I.C., Mountz H., Jacobs T., Rich N., Fish L.J., Noonan D. "Improving the Health of Public Housing Residents Through a Housing Authority and Nursing School Partnership." *Progress in Community Health Partnerships: Research, Education, and Action* 15:1 (2021), 59–64.

References

Aidala, A. A., Wilson, M. G., Shubert, V., Gogolishvili, D., Globerman, J., Rueda, S., Bozack, A. K., Caban, M., & Rourke, S. B. (2016). Housing status, medical care, and health outcomes among people living with HIV/AIDS: A systematic review. *American Journal of Public Health*, *106*(1), e1–e23.

American Association of Colleges of Nursing (AACN). (2008). *The essentials of baccalaureate education for professional nursing practice*. Retrieved December 28, 2019, at https://www.aacnnursing.org/Portals/42/Publications/BaccEssentials08.pdf

Baker, E., Beer, A., Lester, L., Pevalin, D., Whitehead, C., & Bentley, R. (2017). Is housing a health insult? *International Journal of Environmental Research and Public Health, 14*(6), 567.

Bavenko-Mould, Y., Ferguson, K., & Atthill, S. (2016). Neighborhood as community: A qualitative descriptive study of nursing students' experiences of community health nursing. *Nurse Education in Practice, 17,* 223–228.

Biederman, D. J., Callejo-Black, P., Douglas, C., Daeges, M., O'Donohue, H., Brown, A., Olamiji, S. Changes in health and healthcare utilization following eviction from public housing. *Public Health Nursing*.

Biederman, D. J., Hartman, A. M., Felsman, I. C., Mountz, H., Jacobs, T., Rich, N., Fish, L. J., & Noonan, D. (2021). Improving the health of public housing residents through a housing authority and nursing school partnership. *Progress in Community Health Partnerships: Research, Education, and Action, 15*(1), 59–64.

Callejo-Black, P., Biederman, D. J., Douglas, C., & Silberberg, M. (2021). Eviction as a disruptive factor in health care utilization: impact on hospital readmissions and no-show rates. *Journal of Health Care for the Poor and Underserved, 32*(1), 386–396.

Centers for Disease Control and Prevention (CDC). (2019). Cigarette smoking and tobacco use among people of low socioeconomic status. Retrieved from https://www.cdc.gov/tobacco/disparities/low-ses/index.htm

Durham Housing Authority (DHA). (2021). *DHA history 1949–1959*. Retrieved from http://www.durhamhousingauthority.org/about-dha/history/1949–1959/

Goytia, C. N., Todaro-Rivera, L., Brenner, B., Shepard, P., Piedras, V., & Horowitz, C. (2013). Community capacity building: A collaborative approach to designing a training and education model. *Progress in Community Health Partnerships, 7*(3), 291–299. https://doi.org/10.1353/cpr.2013.0031

Mayer, K., Braband, B., & Killen, T. (2017). Exploring collaboration in a community-academic partnership. *Public Health Nursing, 34,* 541–546. https://doi.org/10.1111/phn.12346

Noonan, D., Hartman, A., Briggs, J., & Biederman, D. (2017). Collaborating with public housing residents and staff to improve health: A mixed-methods analysis. *Journal of Community Health Nursing, 34*(4), 203–213. https://doi.org/10.1080/07370016.2017.1369810

Ruel, E., Oakley, D., Wilson, G. E., & Maddox, R. (2010). Is public housing the cause of poor health or a safety net for the unhealthy poor? *Journal of Urban Health*, *87*(5), 827–838.

Singh, A., Daniel, L., Baker, E., & Bentley, R. (2019). Housing disadvantage and poor mental health: A systematic review. *American Journal of Preventive Medicine*, *57*(2), 262–272.

Thompson, C., & Buchner, J. (2013). Meeting baccalaureate public/community health nursing education competencies in nurse-managed wellness center. *Journal of Professional Nursing, 29*(3), 155–162. https://doi.org/10.1016/j.profnurs.2012.04.017

U.S. Census Bureau. (2020). *Quick facts Durham County, NC*. Retrieved from https://www.census.gov/quickfacts/durhamcountynorthcarolina

U.S. Department of Commerce, Bureau of the Census. (1950). *1950 census of population: Preliminary counts*. Report no. series PC-2, no. 10. Retrieved from https://www2.census.gov/library/publications/decennial/1950/pc-02/pc-2-10.pdf

U.S. Department of Housing and Urban Development (HUD). (2016). *Instituting smoke-free public housing*. Retrieved from https://www.hud.gov/sites/documents/SMOKEFREEPHFINALRULE.PDF

Chapter 7

Partnering to Develop Utah's Strategic Plan on Homelessness

Lina Svedin and Jesus N. Valero

The project described in this chapter stemmed from a desire to reduce human suffering associated with homelessness, and contribute in a positive way to the policy environment in Utah, the state in which the researchers live. We believe in evidence-based policy, collaborative governance, and bridging the divide between research and practice. When approached by a policy advocate to support the state in developing a strategic plan on homelessness, we drew on our multidisciplinary experiences and training to develop a plan that would address the healthcare, shelter, and housing needs of homeless individuals and families in Utah, employing a multitude of sources, perspectives, and out-of-state experiences.

The need for a statewide strategic plan crystalized in 2018, when the Utah Legislature mandated the Utah State Homelessness Coordinating Committee (SHCC) to develop a statewide strategic plan on homelessness by October 2019. The research team offered to provide support for this mandated work in partnership with the Division of Housing and Community Development of the Utah Department of Workforce Services, the administrative home for the SHCC. We studied existing research and policies, collected original data, and drafted the state strategic plan over three and a half months, utilizing a methodology that prioritized community collaboration. The drafting process purposely emphasized diverse input, early input, transparency, and open communication. The committee charged with the mandate would consider, revise, and possibly adopt the drafted plan. The research team was given a free hand to suggest the design and execution of the research and drafting process based on their expertise. We kept the adage "nothing about us without us" in mind, as we set out to draft a plan that might impact vulnerable and stigmatized populations, cash-strapped service providers, and hardworking frontline caseworkers in the state for the foreseeable future.

This chapter delineates the process that the research team undertook to develop a strategic plan, including building a partnership with a community organization, our process for studying existing research and connecting with experts, our data collection methods and analysis, the experience in writing the actual strategic plan, and the lessons learned from the entire partnering process. We seek to describe the nuts and bolts of community-engaged strategic planning, with a focus on a full range of needs such as healthcare, housing, and employment services for homeless persons, across a wide range of local conditions.

The community-engaged interdisciplinary research that we were privileged enough to be able to pursue in this project is near and dear to both of us for a number of reasons. First of all, we spend our lives educating, training, and coaching early and mid-career public servants from the public and nonprofit sectors. We give them the very best we have to offer in terms of where current research stands and what theories one can use to make sense of the world, equipping our students with critical analytical tools and habits of mind. We apply for grants to train graduate students to do hands-on research with us and explore topics we feel are critical to building a better functioning and more just society, and both of us care deeply about the communities we come from and the communities we live in. We are both immigrants to Utah but have chosen to make the state our home. We do research on collaboration, community engagement, service provision, accountability, ethics, and marginalized people in societies. Thus, for us, offering to help our state get good information to build the state plan on homelessness was an opportunity to give back to the community we live in by doing something we happen to be particularly good at. The trust, the collaboration, and the partnerships that grew out of our effort to give back far exceeded what we could have hoped for and carried our work and our thinking much further than we anticipated. How we went about forming these partnerships and what that process of drafting the state strategic plan on homelessness in 2019 looked like is what this chapter outlines. Because the process we engaged in was anything but linear and clean-cut, we organize and discuss the dynamic and fluid process of drafting a statewide strategic plan in chronological order through stages.

Stage 1: Getting Asked to Draft the Strategic Plan and Building the Community Partnership
Gaining Access and Developing a Partnership

Two formidable challenges to community-engaged research and research that seeks to influence policy are: (1) most researchers do not have the community connection and credibility that is needed for community partners to seek them out for this type of collaboration; and (2) there is a mismatch between the marching speed with which the world of practice runs and the snail-like speed with which administrative and research approval processes churn in academia. Opportunities to collaborate with community partners are often gone before researchers manage to get approval from institutional review boards to do the research and university offices of sponsored projects to check all the boxes to allow for an actual transfer of money. At least that is the common perception among practitioners and researchers, and all too often it is the sad experience of fledgling collaborative ventures. To be clear, the reason we were successful in conducting the research that had policy impact was that we managed to overcome these two challenges. The ways we overcame these obstacles were: (1) someone acted as a liaison between us and the community partner who had a need; and (2) the University of Utah Office of Sponsored Projects was, by academic standards, incredibly quick and nimble in setting up the contract that allowed us the time and resources to do the project in the short amount of time allowed to the community partner to accomplish it.

As instructors in two professional master's programs, the Master of Public Administration and Master of Public Policy, we enjoy extensive connections and had considerable experience working with practitioners in the field we study. The longevity and prominence of these two degree programs in the local context also bring a certain level of respectability to their instructors, researchers, and graduates who frequently work and lead locally. The initiative to connect us with the community partner came from an alumnus of the Master of Public Administration program who directs a local nonprofit providing services and housing to homeless veterans. The alumnus—an engaged stakeholder on the issue that we were about to study—is respected in the community and is a known advocate with a considerable amount of social capital in Utah's homeless services system. As an active program alumnus, he had a personal and professional relationship with one of us, which made him willing to take the initiative and put some of his social capital on the line to vouch for the quality of work that engaging us could bring to the strategic planning process.

At the outset, and in the presence of the alumnus who served as a liaison, we held an initial meeting with the community partner, the Division of Housing and Community Development of the Utah Department of Workforce Services (the DHCD and community partner from here on). This first meeting was scheduled to iron out what the community partner was looking for, what information it had, what information it needed, and how we as researchers could contribute to that process. This was a meeting for expressing desired ends, objectives, and procedural preferences on behalf of the community partner. It was also a meeting to establish a common language for talking about groups, processes, and data. For us as researchers, it was a dive head-first into a world of practice that is riddled with acronyms, personal relationships, disparate data collection points, and divergent data organization, and an attempt to establish what the community partner was hoping to do with data eventually. After a lot of active listening on our part, some parameters were set in terms of what we as a research team thought we could do, how we might go about doing the work, and what points on the community partner's wish list we understood to be the greatest priority. We huddled following this meeting and came to an agreement about what we thought the needs and interests of our potential community partner were as well as the research design that was both ethically responsive and feasible under the time constraints (we were given approximately three months).

A formal proposal was drafted on how we thought the work to complete a strategic plan could be done. The proposal contained information on our scientific approach (i.e., review of literature and best practices, analysis of existing data, and collection of new data through focus groups and interviews) as well as our proposed timeline for conducting the work. Included with the proposal was a draft budget of the resources needed to carry out the work, including stipends for the researchers and graduate assistants, and resources for organizing and hosting community forums across the state. We submitted the proposal and budget to the community partner for consideration and feedback, and they were returned without comments or concerns. Our community partner served as a liaison between us, the research team, and the State Homeless Coordinating Committee that had the statutory responsibility for developing the plan and needed to sign off on our proposal and budget. Our next step was to approach our institutional grant management office to begin drafting a contract.

Getting Formal Approval and Contracting with the State

As the flagship university of Utah located in Salt Lake City, the University of Utah has many contracts and collaborations with different state offices, foundations, and other entities. More important for the purposes of this interdisciplinary community-engaged research, however, the College of Social and Behavioral Science grant management staff had previously set up contracts with the community partner on earlier projects for a different college department. Consequently, when the research team approached the college grant management office, the staff had a model on which to base the cost estimates and contract language. This was critical as the timeline for the project was quite short by academic standards, and the project was set to start virtually immediately if the project and funding was approved by the State Homelessness Coordinating Committee. Once the university prepared a draft of the contract and budget, we shared the documents with our community partner who reviewed and then submitted them to the State Homelessness Coordinating Committee for their final review and approval.

We were invited by the community partner to present our proposed way of collecting information and drafting the Utah strategic plan on homelessness to the State Homelessness Coordinating Committee three weeks after our initial conversation with the community partner. We prepared a short PowerPoint presentation and we were allotted approximately ten minutes to present. At the committee meeting, the community partner organization expressed its support for the proposal and presented the cost of the contract. The committee voted to approve our proposal and our budget at the end of the meeting and no questions were posed by the committee. We then moved quickly to begin the project.

Stage 2: Getting Acquainted with the Literature, Developing Key Research Documents, and Understanding the Local Context
Reviewing Existing Research and Other Strategic Plans

In order to make sure that we as researchers were up-to-date on current trends, ideas, and changes in the world of homeless service provision, we needed to take a deep dive into all the key resource materials we could locate. We needed to do this for several reasons. First, we wanted to make sure that the plan we drafted was well grounded in best practices and current national thinking on homelessness. Second, a review of existing knowledge was important to maintaining credibility and securing the confidence of local experts who participated in the research process—a group that is frequently skeptical of what academics can bring to a world that they, the experts, know so well. Knowing our stuff was an essential first strand in what was going to be a carefully twined rope of trust, which would hopefully be strong enough to swing us through some treacherous political jungles at high speed.

We began by conducting an extensive search of relevant scholarly articles from 2009 to 2019, focused on research that covered collaborative governance and homeless programs. We focused our search to the last ten years as we were most interested in cutting-edge thinking on homelessness. We also searched for and read existing state and federal policies and reports. Specifically, we reviewed reports on homelessness produced by the U.S. Interagency Council on Homelessness and the Department of Housing and Urban Development. We also studied strategic plans on homelessness from states in the Western Census region as Utah falls within this region and we were interested in cases most similar in geographic composition and location. After our study of this gathered information, we conducted content analyses and did a thematic clustering of the material such as causes of homelessness, existing approaches to homeless policy, and factors contributing to a reduction in homelessness.

Developing Our Research Documents

Based on our review of the literature and expectations set by our community partner in terms of the goals and objectives of the strategic plan, we sought to develop a draft focus group and interview facilitation guide that we would ultimately use to conduct semistructured conversations with community stakeholders. We settled on adopting Ansell and Gash's (2008) model of collaborative governance as a guide to developing a truly collaborative statewide strategic plan because their framework was comprehensive and the result of a thorough analysis of existing research on collaboration governance. We also considered the amount of time that we would have with any community stakeholder and felt it would be most appropriate to stick with the best practice of keeping any engagement to no more than one hour. All of this then helped in identifying four key areas of interest needing input from stakeholders: (1) conditions in the community, (2) how to improve the process of working together and coordinating action, (3) how to measure impact and benchmarks, and lastly, (4) other topics that the stakeholders felt were important that had not been addressed by our questions and prompting—with three to four relevant questions in each area. Our goal was to obtain direct feedback and ideas on how to build a plan that would achieve collaborative governance on the issue of homeless policy in the state. We ran this preliminary list of topic areas and questions by our community partner who then agreed to the content and focus areas.

Engaging the Local and State Experts and Others

We also recognized the importance of involving, early on, key leaders of the stakeholder groups who had great influence on how the plan would be received, who held important information, and who possessed resources that the plan would rely on to get the job done. Doing so would also help us obtain buy-in, get leaders on the same page about what we were proposing to do, and obtain their feedback on our proposed process. Thus, we felt it was appropriate and advantageous to hold an initial meeting with these leaders, including state officials, nonprofit managers, and other key community leaders.

We purposefully organized a meeting with the leadership of the three Utah Continuum of Care (CoC) networks[1]—Salt Lake County, Mountainland, and Balance of State, the community partner

---

1. The Continuum of Care structure is superordinate to and helps coordinate efforts among the local homeless coordinating committees. Many of the CoCs are the receiving organizations for federal funding for homelessness that they then distribute or build projects with, drawing on the local homeless coordinating committees that are included geographically in individual CoC areas.

organization, and others that our community partner felt should be present. The healthcare needs of homeless individuals are frequently complex, costly, and acute (APA, 2020; CDC, 2020). Part of the U.S. Department of Housing and Urban Development's strategy to mitigate homelessness builds on these Continuum of Care networks (HUD, 2020) to work together as a coordinated service web in addressing underlying issues of homelessness, such as chronic health conditions, substance use disorders, and unaddressed mental health needs (APA, 2020). These organizations and the individuals that represent them thereby occupy important coordinating functions and make key funding allocation decisions in the state homeless service system.

We ran this initial meeting exactly the way that we would run the subsequent focus groups and tested the content of the facilitation guide we had drafted with these state and local leaders. We aimed to show the leaders a proof of concept of our focus group process, demonstrate our leadership and facilitation skills to inventory their values (as representations of deeper veins of values, conflicts, and priorities that were out there in the communities of stakeholders), and bring to the surface and recognize some of the values and value conflicts raised in creating a statewide strategic plan.

The discussion helped us determine the number of questions that could effectively be covered in a group, how to document the discussion effectively, how much to moderate the discussion, and what roles each of us would need to take. The discussion also helped uncover a series of core values that stakeholder leaders were committed to and prioritized, as well as some of the power bases from which they operated. Having the leaders become aware of and recognize the contribution of other leaders and the resources, access, and power they brought to the table was key to the leaders committing their power, access, and resources to the research team as we set out to do the work the community partner organization had contracted us to do.

As a research team, we would be heavily dependent on these leaders to organize the focus groups, get the appropriate representatives to show up for meetings, lend their credibility and know-how to us to overcome local skepticism about state-level efforts in this policy area, and get a mix of types of stakeholders at the table (a balance was unlikely but we wanted to make sure the focus groups were as inclusive as possible). Because each CoC network has a specific geographic jurisdiction, we asked each for its assistance in coordinating a focus group in their communities. For example, the Balance of State CoC network in Utah is comprised primarily of rural Utah and one of their coordinators assisted us in organizing focus groups at the local coordinating committee level.

In addition to local and state leaders, we also sought to connect with other experts in the field operating in other states or at the federal level of homeless services, whom we already had professional connections with or had been referred to by experts we knew. All of them were willing to share their knowledge and insights with us once we explained what we had been tasked to do and what information we were looking for, but not every expert we contacted got back to us in time for us to incorporate their insights into our analysis. We were, however, successful in interviewing the regional representatives for Utah from the U.S. Interagency Council on Homelessness as well as the U.S. Department of Housing and Urban Development. These conversations were particularly fruitful for understanding the federal perspective on Utah's challenges, needs, and possible solutions.

Stage 3: Traveling across the State to Meet Local Stakeholders
Organizing the Focus Groups

As public policy scholars, we insisted that those affected have input early on in the policy development process, not after the policy options had been crafted. In policymaking, in general, stakeholder impact is frequently minimized by involving groups late, having them react to a preset agenda or only giving them the option of getting behind or rejecting a fully developed plan that is up for a vote. While we knew the importance of early input from stakeholders, figuring out how to facilitate that and what it would look like in our rather condensed research schedule of approximately three months was a challenge.

Having proved to the leaders of key stakeholder organizations in this policy area that the focus group process was productive and that we were appropriately skilled in facilitating such discussions, we split the work of organizing the focus groups and garnering support to conduct them. One of us worked with the Balance of State CoC and its coordinator to pick dates to hold focus groups with each local coordinating committee and identify the types of participants the research team was interested in having represented in the focus group while keeping the number of participants manageable. The other person worked on getting graduate research assistants together to staff the focus groups over the next six weeks and to support the analysis of the focus group materials.

From a methodological point of view, we preferred a smaller number of participants (eight to ten per group); however, the CoC representatives helping pull the focus groups together and coordinating with local representatives foresaw that a larger number would be necessary (twenty to twenty-five). They anticipated that there would be a great amount of interest in contributing to the process and some localities had a large number of engaged stakeholders. A compromise was made to aim for twelve to fifteen, with our team offering to be flexible if a larger than expected number of stakeholders wanted to participate locally. While we were aware of the challenges that facilitating a conversation among twenty persons would pose, we consciously chose to be accommodating to the realities of circumstances, to make the work for the representatives as easy as possible, and not come across as insisting on unrealistic and overly rigid research methods—things that often keep academia from being consulted on real-world issues in public policy. We were instead open to and willing to rise to the occasion, bringing our very best efforts and game to the process to bridge the gap between the ideal and the situation at hand. It was important to get the focus groups done and to have as diverse a set of participants as possible. We also did the cold calculation that attrition would draw the actual number of participants down for each planned focus group.

In the end, our research team conducted fourteen focus groups across the state of Utah over six weeks. A total of 170 individuals representing nonprofit organizations, government, citizens, and other stakeholders participated in these groups. Specifically, focus groups were organized with twelve out of Utah's thirteen Local Homeless Coordinating Committees (LHCCs). The focus groups took place in spaces where the Local Homeless Coordinating Committees normally met. Our team also conducted one focus group specifically with frontline staff of homeless services providers within Salt Lake County—the largest CoC in Utah in terms of providers, homeless individuals, and funding—to get a better sense of how that CoC's service provision system was experienced by those who worked within it on a daily basis. The Salt Lake CoC had just reorganized its service provision system and its governance structure in order to improve functionality and overcome some existing challenges, and we wanted to hear from those working in the system what these challenges looked like so they could be considered in the overall state plan.

Growing the Research Team and Training on the Road

As dates and locations for local focus groups were coming in, we were keenly aware that we were not going to be able to do fourteen to sixteen focus groups across the state over six weeks without additional help. We understood that at a minimum, we would need two or three team members per focus group with one person facilitating the discussion, one person taking notes, and another assisting with the coordination of the meeting (i.e., welcoming guests, answering questions, and providing general support) and taking secondary notes. We had prioritized ease of scheduling and participation, so the CoC representatives were booking focus group meetings to coincide with local coordinating committee meetings that were scheduled to be held in the upcoming month. This also meant that the focus groups would need to run during the day, sometimes in very far-away corners of the state without public transportation, freeways, or many options in terms of catering. The scheduling of some of the focus groups meant that the team running the focus group would need to drive for hours, sleep in a hotel, and then get up and go get catered coffee and snacks or lunch before starting the group.

We recruited graduate students from the professional master's degree programs we are engaged with and from the Department of Political Science at the University of Utah. We considered students who were former research or graduate assistants, students with interest or professional background in homeless policy, students who expressed an interest in developing research skills, and students who were available over the summer months. A total of ten graduate students responded to our call for participation.

To begin, we held an orientation session with the students during which we provided them with background on the state statute requiring the development of the strategic plan, the current state of homeless policy and services in Utah, our plan for conducting the research and timeline, and the important role that they as graduate students would play in the process. We provided the students with a guide on best practices for participating in and conducting focus groups. As an opportunity to observe how a focus group would be conducted, we invited the students to attend our first community focus group as a training session. In addition, for the first couple of focus groups, students only assisted with taking detailed notes, recording the session, and coordinating of the meeting. Once students felt comfortable and had plenty of experience observing focus groups, we gave them an opportunity to lead and facilitate a session. We continued to provide coaching to the students as sessions progressed over the six weeks.

The graduate students turned out to be an extraordinary resource, being very quick learners, socially adept, and very capable. As research leaders we felt comfortable enough in the last phase of the focus groups to send the graduate students out on their own, as a team, to conduct a number of focus groups that we could not make as the scheduling unfolded and prior commitments collided. For one of the focus group days, we literally had three focus groups scheduled in completely disparate parts of the state, and in order to get them all done, we had to divide and conquer. Recruiting graduate students from very relevant professional programs (public policy and public administration) and some with research experience or interest in homeless policy, turned out to be beneficial as they required little training and onboarding. Our ability to also recruit students from various professional backgrounds, from law enforcement and from the nonprofit sector for example, was also an asset in obtaining their feedback and perspectives on local homeless policy. We benefited from the thoughtful ideas that students had for solutions to our state's challenges on homelessness and from their astute observations from the field. From our teacher perspective, we enjoyed the opportunity to offer our students a professional development opportunity and mentorship. We were fortunate enough to not encounter any significant issues or challenges in engaging our students in the research process—they were all professional, dedicated, and dependable.

Stage 4: Writing the Strategic Plan

We conducted an inductive thematic analysis of the focus group responses, largely organized by the set of questions the discussion had centered on. This allowed us to highlight common themes across Utah's homeless services and locales. Service gaps, needed resources, core values, and what was working successfully were some of the key pieces that came out of that analysis. We learned, for example, that increased access to case management services was key to effectively addressing the multidimensional needs of those experiencing homelessness, including referrals to healthcare and other community supports. We also identified a number of institutional barriers, challenges, and needs that, if addressed, would make the homeless services system as a whole work better. A remaining and important part of our analysis was understanding Utah's performance in terms of eradicating homelessness and how it compared to other similar states.

Thus, another segment of the analysis that went into the strategic plan on homelessness included lots of thoughts about how Utah as a state as well as individual localities performed compared to other states in the United States and relative to federal measures of system performance. Our conversations with representatives from the U.S. Department of Housing and Urban Development (HUD) and the U.S. Interagency Council on Homelessness (USICH) were helpful in understanding how the federal government understood performance measurement and improvement, specifically the realization that benchmarks were not pre-scribed. We knew that figuring out measures and benchmarks of perfor-mance would be a potential challenge as our focus group conversations had little to say about this matter.

The team also thought proactively about the policy initiatives and pri-ority changes we were drafting, and what implementation would need to look like in order for proposed changes to be rolled out effectively and with intended results. We then took the step to write a set of recommen-dations that were in alignment with the needs and challenges that we observed across the state and that were identified through our thematic analysis of focus group data.

When, after much effort, our team submitted the draft plan and the community partner organization immediately scheduled two three-hour conference calls to discuss the draft, it was clear that revisions would be needed. On the one hand, there were elements we as researchers felt comfortable saying and supporting based on what had been voiced by stakeholders that had participated in the process. On the other hand, there were specific and tangible policy performance targets that the community partner organization members sensed that the head of their organization would be looking for and that they would need in order to utilize the strategic plan as the basis for funding allocation to local coordinating committees. The community partner organization wanted numerical performance measures and corresponding benchmarks to measure and report progress toward reaching system improvement.

In a sense, the community partner staff was asking for a merged deductive and inductive plan. The DHCD wanted the Utah statewide plan on homelessness to be responsive to state officials expecting concrete performance measures and benchmarks, but also respect and draw on the work that local committees and the Utah CoCs had been doing and had established data reporting on. The challenge of balancing the desire for the best possible current data, looking toward future needs, and the reality of the limited capacity and resources service providers have to dedicate to data collection and data reporting is not uncommon in the world of policy development. The conflict between parsimony and detail is real when so many of the details are context-based, even as we grapple with homelessness as a condition across the state. We heard the community partner organization's additional needs and desires and were able to express doubt as to the wisdom of setting specific numerical targets; we noted that no indications, inductively or deductively, were available to help our team set benchmarks that would not to some extent feel arbitrary. Recognizing these challenges, the community partner nevertheless sent us off to revise the draft to better meet their needs and expectations.

Rewriting the first draft was as much a battle of massive information reorganization as it was a mental struggle for the research team to stretch to the very edges of what they were willing to say with authority. Much of what was available in terms of best practices from states were highly localized solutions, experimental approaches, and pilot tested programs, so there was not a lot that could be directly transferred as well-supported evidence-based policy. The federal perspective was comprehensive and informative but only suggestive and mildly worded, which did not make for a strong authoritative voice on best practices. The team carried those pilot programs that had had some success and were being adopted by some other entities into Utah's draft plan. The team also tried to read between the lines to get what the federal organizations were really suggesting by reading prior plans and suggestions and seeing where the federal perspective seemed to be shifting. The team took those tendencies at the federal level to be a soft target for policy performance, knowing that great variation between states made it tenuous to generalize across policy environments.

Finally, virtually no state or the federal government organization had the type of numerical policy performance targets that the community partner was looking for. In fact, most states had moved away from setting specific numerical or even percentage change goals, recognizing that the policy area is very dynamic, fluid, and locally conditioned. As a team we struggled with this as it was clear that our community partner wanted very tangible goals and performance measures that could be assessed and compared from year to year. Wracking our brains, rereading other state plans and reports, we finally decided to speak truth to power and assert that selecting a numerical target or benchmark to hit each year as a measure of good performance was something that the team was recommending against. It was not supported by other states' work and had at times been found by other states to actually reduce policy effectiveness. In the end, Utah's plan contained performance measures and a suggested target improvement rate for individual localities. The plan, however, measured percentage performance improvements from the situation in the locality at the adoption of the statewide strategic plan, rather than an arbitrary comparable performance improvement number based on other states or localities.

Rewriting the first draft in order to map and align Utah's emerging plan conceptually and methodologically to the federal plan on homelessness also ended up being a feat of mental gymnastics. At one point, one of us had the entire draft of the report printed out, cut into sections, numbered, reorganized, and taped together in long rolls all around the office as a way to pull the new version together without losing any vital information. The other team member received the reorganized document and went through it to condense, simplify, and clarify the logic of the plan. We also footnoted a lot of the data, methodology, and comparisons that were the foundation for the plan. The revised plan was set to be presented to the State Homelessness Coordinating Committee a week later. The community partner organization dedicated some personnel hours to copyediting the second draft and did an initial report layout before the draft was circulated to the committee members in advance of the meeting where we were expected to present the plan. The draft plan was also published for public comment at this point and twelve comments were submitted electronically during this period. While there were few public comments, several of them were from key political stakeholders as well as key service providers with considerable experience and knowledge about the homeless provider system in Utah and other states. Comments were predominantly focused on requesting greater clarity on the organization of the document and on the importance of pointing to differences in needs across communities, particularly urban versus rural.

We used PowerPoint slides to summarize how the information in the draft plan had been collected and compared. The presentation to the committee also included how Utah's plan mapped onto the federal plan, and what the main takeaways and priorities in the plan were. The floor was opened to questions and the committee asked to have time to review the full draft in advance of a vote to adopt the plan at the next meeting. In the meantime, our team was asked by the committee to simplify the report, make it less wordy, add more pictures, and make it easy to navigate visually. While researchers are rarely asked to make their points less wordy by academic audiences, we heard the need for a busy policymaking audience to be able to quickly navigate and comprehend the plan, so we went back to the drawing board again and cut many explanations, justifications, points of comparison, and description from the body of the plan. One of us also went through every public comment and incorporated as much of the feedback and suggestions as possible in the final draft of the plan. We were keenly aware that in order for the plan to be adopted and implemented effectively, those who had contributed to the process and had specific feedback on the draft needed to be heard and see evidence of that in the revised version of the plan.

The community partner wanted a set of action items identified in the final version of the plan, including which organizations or leaders would be responsible for leading the work on these action items. Because this detailed implementation map and action item rollout required in-depth knowledge of areas or responsibilities and compatibility of resources and missions, we did a first draft of this action item implementation map but asked the community partner organization to help identify what organization would be the most appropriate to lead on each item as well as which item would require collaboration between multiple actors. This identification process took place over conference calls with several public servants and experts included to ensure appropriateness of fit. The community partner organization finally reviewed the text for clarity, proofread the language, and provided a professional layout of the third and final draft of the Utah strategic plan on homelessness. This final draft of the plan was submitted to the committee for its review and the strategic plan was approved and adopted in October of 2019.

Lessons Learned along the Way

As a research team fortunate enough to develop a reciprocal relationship with a community organization to help support and impact policy, we learned a great deal. These lessons clearly pertain to the project discussed in this chapter but we think they have wider implications for effectiveness in interdisciplinary community-engaged research on housing and health.

• *Being clear, succinct, and practical is key.* Busy policymakers need information, plans, and reports that are easy to digest, clear, and succinct. Our first draft of the strategic plan contained more information than was preferred, at least in the way we had presented it. Our community partner wanted goals, measures, and benchmarks upfront with more details of implementation in later sections. They preferred that all other details, such as the methodology and our process for calculating the measures and benchmarks, be included as an appendix. We also learned that policymakers and particularly advocates want key points highlighted in a visually accessible way that allows them to get the gist quickly and that helps them speak intelligently about how and where they stand on the issue.

• *Groups under threat pull together.* Consensus in groups that are under a great deal of scrutiny and political pressure is more important than the details of the issue they are agreeing on. Once everyone in the State Homeless Coordinating Committee (SHCC) agreed that they probably needed some help coming up with the strategic plan, it was less important how or who was providing that support. Moreover, once we had been vetted by individuals in the community partner organization whom the SHCC trusted it was not difficult for the SHCC to come to a consensus to approve the specific support contracted. Being academics with research experience in the topic, resources available to help us achieve the work, and a genuine willingness to be a true collaborative partner, we believe, helped secure the support of key stakeholders, but the group dynamics of the SHCC played an independent reinforcing role.

• *People want to matter.* What happens in rural areas is often experienced by local organizers and public servants as unimportant to policymakers located in the state capital. The disconnect to conditions and challenges in rural and low-density communities is not just geographic. We found that data were missing, perceptions about local conditions were inaccurate, funding was scarce, collaboration challenging, and disempowerment palpable. The profound gratitude that our team was met with, simply for traveling to the locations in rural Utah where many of the LHCCs met, was tremendous and actively supported a collaborative spirit in the focus groups. The legwork that we as a research team did to meet stakeholder groups on their turf, where they were, and on their time schedule, paid off in spades in terms of the work LHCCs did to pull participants into the focus groups and the valuable data that we were able to collect. This ultimately helped us draft a plan that included voices and perspectives from urban, suburban, and rural areas—a plan for all of Utah.

• *In interdisciplinary community-engaged research, how you research matters as much as what you produce.* The level of acceptance and even excitement around the Utah strategic plan on homelessness that many stakeholders exhibited when the adopted plan was discussed at the Utah Homeless Summit in October 2019 should be attributed to the fact that stakeholders could see their own perspective and input reflected in the final plan. The effort that went into collecting input; honestly identifying themes related to challenges, resource needs, and what was already working around the state; and translating that into realistic and practical steps forward, is what created buy-in from the local community stakeholders that would be needed to implement the plan. As researchers, our commitment to collecting as complete a body of information as possible, without skewing the input process toward already privileged voices, and reporting back honestly what we saw, reflected our commitment to speaking truth to power. Prioritizing transparency, collaboration, and community input characterized how we went about collecting that information. We believe that *how* we went about gathering information for the plan was just as important to gaining and sustaining stakeholder trust as the actual actions and solutions we proposed in the final drafted plan.

• *Modeling best practices.* The importance of walking the walk, not just talking the talk, was highlighted a number of times during the data collection for and drafting of the state strategic plan on homelessness. First, we realized that we needed to convince the community partner and other key leaders that focus groups were not only a valuable tool but a necessity to get the type of information we would need to build the plan. In order to do this, we conducted the first focus group with the very people who would need to buy into the proposed research plan. We modeled in real-time just how valuable a focus group process is for uncovering values undergirding positions, perceptions, system functionality, and desired ends. Second, we had a desire to "bright-spot" and to avoid falling into the trap of saying that nothing is working or that the people who had made substantive investments and efforts under the current system were doing a bad job. By listening to what stakeholders thought was working well and what they would like to keep in the current system, as well as doing an inventory of successful practices around the country, we managed to preserve the pride and hope that current successes carried for those working in the system. Finally, our willingness as researchers to adjust to the schedule and conditions that practitioners face every day was part of modeling that a successful academic and community partnership can be formed to conduct vital and impactful research for practice. Modeling how a community-academic partnership can work for the community partner, those that participated in the focus groups, and the graduate students who were trained, is one part of a larger effort to generate high-quality interdisciplinary community-engaged research; not just with regard to homelessness but many of the complex and persistent social challenges of our lifetime.

• *Bridging research and practice.* The struggle over benchmarks and performance measures in this community-engaged study is reflective of a common but persistent conflict between the desire to be certain and the world being complicated and frequently in flux. Everyone who engaged in the strategic planning process wanted the best possible plan and wanted to alleviate the problems associated with homelessness. How each stakeholder thinks about and assesses a good plan and what making progress on alleviating homelessness looks like, however, varies a great deal depending on where one sits and what one's experience has been. As researchers we tended to think Utah compared well to other states or even an aggregate of states that may be relevant. Localities, however, saw the most use and significance in comparing their own performance to their prior performance, not compared to any other locality, as they were painfully aware of the differences in strengths and weaknesses among local coordinating committees. The community partner, the DHCD, thought in terms of comparing Utah's performance on homelessness to other innovative and effective states but also comparing themselves to what the federal guidelines for best practices and good performance looked like. For researchers, evidence, preferably large amounts of evidence across cases, make a solid basis for projecting trends, forming expectations, and possibly measuring performance and outcomes. Innovating in terms of measures of outcomes and setting performance benchmarks or policy targets seemed reckless and unfair without substantial evidence that this performance could and should be expected of stakeholders. Nevertheless, the need to have a target number, some tangible way of measuring and showing progress, toward a set of policy goals was really important to the community partner, who saw a need to clearly signal policy directions and a policy movement pace that would keep a diverse set of stakeholders engaged and accountable. In the end, the compromise on benchmarks and performance measures that was included in the plan was a compromise between these different needs and understandings.

• *Institutional support pays dividends.* From prior research experiences at our university, we have learned the value and importance of having the backing, support, and the resources from our institution to make doing research a smoother process. We benefited greatly from a grants management office team that was responsive, had experience, and that was willing to help and answer questions from the initial contracting process to the final days of reconciling our spending account. Our ability to tap into graduate student resources in our programs is also a symptom of an institution of higher learning that values the inclusion of students in research projects. When we approached our department leadership about recruiting students and then hiring them, we received an overwhelming yes! We felt that having this level of institutional support helped us stay focused on the final goal: writing the state's first strategic plan on homelessness.

Conclusion

In sum, the authors learned a great deal through this experience about the process of developing a strategic plan for a state to reduce the incidence of homelessness. From the beginning, we realized that the state and our community partner were 100 percent invested in a process that would help stakeholders understand the current conditions of our state, ways of improving the system, measures for benchmarking progress, and a collective mission and vision for all stakeholders to buy into. While the process was quite time-sensitive, the active engagement of our community partner, the incredible support of our institutional grant management office, the inclusion and training of graduate students, and our genuine willingness to listen, adjust, and learn all proved crucial to the success of the research and planning process. In the end, the strategic plan was adopted in October 2019 and was officially rolled out at that year's state conference on homelessness—where providers, advocates, and community leaders had an opportunity to hear from state leadership about the plan and discuss its value and implementation.

References

American Psychological Association (APA). (2020). Health and homelessness. Retrieved April 1, 2020, from https://www.apa.org/pi/ses/resources/publications/homelessness-health

Ansell, C., & Gash, A. (2008). Collaborative governance in theory and practice. *Journal of Public Administration Research and Theory*, *18*(4), 543–571.

Centers for Disease Control and Prevention (CDC). (2020). Homelessness as a public health law issue: Selected resources. Retrieved April 1, 2020, from https://www.cdc.gov/phlp/publications/topic/resources/resources-homelessness.html

State of Utah Strategic Plan on Homelessness. (2019). Retrieved June 8, 2021, from https://jobs.utah.gov/housing/homelessness/shcc/documents/homelessnessstrategicplan.pdf

U.S. Department of Housing and Urban Development (HUD). (2020). Continuum of care program. Retrieved April 1, 2020, from https://www.hud.gov/hudprograms/continuumofcare

Utah Workforce Services Code §35A-8-601 (2019).

Chapter 8

A View from the Intersection

Mina Silberberg

Health in the United States is shockingly bad. Compared to other industrialized, high-wealth nations, we show up poorly on measures of life expectancy (lowest), infant mortality (highest), obesity, and more (Papinacolas, Woskie, & Jha, 2018). Arguably, some of these poor outcomes can be laid at the feet of a healthcare system that, while boasting of short wait times to see a specialist and sophisticated medical technology, has fewer physicians per capita than the average for similar countries and leaves 10 percent of its population without access to even basic healthcare (Papinacolas, Woskie, & Jha, 2018). It has become clear, however, that the greatest contributors to health status are what have been termed social *drivers* of health (SDoH).

The impact of housing as a social driver of health is well illustrated by the chapters in this volume. The case studies present the views of residents of Baton Rouge on how neighborhood conditions factor into wellness, the contribution of homelessness to poor health that spurred Medicaid to pay for tenancy support services, the health impacts of code enforcement, and the difficulty of managing HIV/AIDS when residing in communities in which that condition is stigmatized. And these are but some of the ways in which housing drives health.

However, the reality of the relationship between a social condition like housing and health is more complex than what is implied by the label of "social driver"—phrasing that suggests the simple causal diagram x → y that is often taught in introductory research classes. For starters, the relationship between housing and health is not unidirectional, but bidirectional, with mental illness, for example, contributing to the conditions of homelessness and institutionalization that tenancy support services are trying to reverse.

That bidirectionality is only the beginning of the complexity. As chapters 2 and 3 demonstrate, housing and health—and the relationship between them—interact with a larger set of contextual and individual-level forces, including religion, social stigma, social connectedness, isolation and division, racism, natural disasters, the economy, policing, and more. The history of Baton Rouge and the theoretical framework provided in chapter 3 to explain its traumatic effects suggest one more layer of complexity—the ongoing legacy and cumulative effects of historical choices on the present. Trauma, in particular, can affect not just an individual but an entire community, and shapes multiple generations over time through its impact on epigenetics, psychological well-being, and social systems. Moreover, structural factors that create trauma—such as racial exclusion—are often at the root of diverse systemic and policy decisions that compound adversity for individuals and for society as a whole. A striking example is the dependence of poor, primarily Black, people in North Baton Rouge on the Earl K. Long Medical Center. The community's lack of material resources, their residential concentration in North Baton Rouge, and the lack of other hospital and behavioral healthcare services in that part of town have their roots in structural racism. Taken together, these conditions mean that the state's decision to close the medical center left residents without hospital or behavioral health services, compounding the community's challenges and dramatically decreasing its resources for addressing them.

Health disparities, as described in this volume, provide us with an important lens on the complex interaction among social factors and health. Regional disparities, such as the differences in HIV prevalence between the Deep South and the rest of the country, indicate a missed opportunity for health improvement. Racial health disparities indicate a context of injustice that must be redressed—a point that is made with particular power by chapter 3's explication of the ways in which racism has contributed to trauma and poor health in Baton Rouge. The research on health disparities and their root causes provides one more body of evidence indicating that health improvement efforts will have limited success if the social drivers of health (with all their complexity) are not addressed. Indeed, it is this realization that has led to the investment of Medicaid in tenancy support services, the development and use of health impact assessments, the funding of research on environmental and social factors at the Duke University School of Nursing, and the decision of the Robert Wood Johnson Foundation to invest heavily in supporting an intersectoral Culture of Health.

To the daunting task of addressing SDoH we bring interdisciplinary community-engaged research (ICEnR). Readers might be forgiven for thinking that the authors of this volume have developed a case of hubris. What would make us think that ICEnR can play the role of David relative to the Goliath of interconnected social, physical, and health factors just described?

This work makes no pretense of slaying the giant on its own, but history suggests that ICEnR has a role to play. To a large extent, the beauty of ICEnR is the fact that it readily lends itself to supporting and enhancing the impact of other efforts that must be made to tackle our social ills—community organizing, cultural change, systems change, policy reform, and so on. ICEnR is designed to encourage the use of research to support and amplify such endeavors. In Alabama, ICEnR is accelerating efforts to reduce the stigma of HIV/AIDS in the faith community. Peer leaders there apply their training to participation in research and also to advocacy; and they mentor the next generation of peer leaders. In the case of the tenancy support services (TSS) study described in chapter 4, the team's research was inspired by policy change resulting from years of advocacy; in turn, that research is contributing to expansion of and changes in housing services. In that case and in Memphis (chapter 5), collaboration is both capitalizing on and amplifying (even expanding) the roles of researchers and community partners. In Durham (chapter 6), community-academic collaboration on a grant proposal that was not funded still resulted in increased police patrols requested by the community. These cases show the chinks in the mesh of Goliath's armor—the places where multiple actors, working together, can insert themselves. Just as interaction among adverse social conditions compounds their effects, so can interaction among efforts to improve health and social well-being create compounded advantage.

So, what specifically are the advantages that ICEnR brings to this endeavor? We have just described one—the potential to move research results off of the library shelf into the arena of action, creating collaborations that compound the benefits of both research and praxis. This work can transform the potential for code enforcement to change lives in Memphis or for medical funding to be spent effectively in a nonmedical arena in Durham.

Another advantage of ICEnR is the potential to raise up the importance of SDoH, as was done by community residents in Baton Rouge who addressed health in terms of its relationship to jobs, social connection, and resources. Recognition of this reality does not just improve our academic explanations of health and health disparities. It has direct consequences for allocation of resources and priority-setting. It is not only Medicaid that has decided to invest in housing in recognition of its effect on its bottom line, but also healthcare systems like Le Bonheur in Memphis. As the Memphis case also shows, demonstrating the health impacts of enforcing specific housing codes can augment the intensity and breadth of political will for enforcement.

Another advantage of ICEnR is the ways in which it strengthens our capacity to "get it right." This assertion raises the question of what "right" means. As noted by Wallerstein and Duran (2017), different approaches to engaged research are associated with different understandings of the nature of knowledge. Nonetheless, these approaches share a rejection of the idea of the objective all-knowing researcher and a belief that inquiry utilizing both research *and* experiential knowledge helps us align our actions with our goals and values. Knowledge is enriched through engagement. The benefits of ICEnR for "getting it right" are illustrated in this volume by such varied results as the expanded understanding of health offered by Baton Rouge residents, the role of the advocate in defining an important research question for the TSS team, and the role of the same team's consumer advisory council in highlighting the triangular relationship among TSS providers, consumers, and landlords. In Memphis, it required housing and public health expertise *and* academic and community expertise to accurately screen, scope, assess, recommend, and report. In Alabama, interdisciplinary researchers representing medicine, clinical research, public health, and psychology brought varied expertise to the study of life with HIV/AIDS; they were further helped in understanding that reality by their partnership with people living with HIV/AIDS and their service providers. In Utah, the state's desire for numerical policy performance targets clashed with the researchers' belief that there was lack of evidence supporting such metrics and that their use had even been damaging in other communities. Extensive and honest communication about this issue resulted in the state focusing on improvement from baseline rather than adopting arbitrary performance benchmarks.

Another advantage of engaged research is its potential to repair social relations. When the social conditions contributing to poor health include distrust and stigma (particularly well-represented in chapter 2) or exclusion and power imbalance (as exemplified in the history of Baton Rouge in chapter 3), ICEnR is not just a means of figuring out the solution, but part of the solution itself. Engaged research helps to redress power imbalances by highlighting the value of the knowledge and voices of people who have been marginalized, augmenting the resources that they have at their disposal to influence decision-making, and amplifying their actions. In fact, in Durham, public housing residents have become teachers of nursing students and are being paid for some of that work, as well as for working as lay health advisors (chapter 6). By creating new relationships of trust and mutual support, engaged research helps to redress the corrosive effects of distrust, social division, and isolation. Even though the TSS researchers in chapter 4 primarily partnered with a policy advocate (with less intensive engagement with individuals receiving services), her perceived legitimacy and standing in decision-making arenas was enhanced by the partnership, thereby strengthening her ability to advocate for the needs of those experiencing homelessness.

While these advantages of ICEnR are compelling, it is a challenging endeavor. George Mugoya and his colleagues in chapter 2 remind us that people vary in personality and temperament—a challenge for all collaborative work. Collaboration can benefit from this diversity (we need both Executors and Refiners to get things done and done well) but it can also be damaged by resulting conflict and misunderstanding. Moreover, ICEnR adds flash points in the form of differences in skills, language, and perspective—ranging from what "CDC" means to conflicting priorities about how to spend one's time. Chapter 7 on Utah highlights two key differences between academics and policymakers. While academics tend to favor extensive research projects requiring a long timeline, policymakers generally need information gathering to be done quickly. At the end of that process, academics favor nuanced conclusions and a high bar for evidence, while policymakers seek certainty and the ability to quickly respond to the demands of key constituencies.

ICEnR faces challenges not only from internal team dynamics, but also from the external environment. In one such example in chapter 4, the inclusion of a policy advocate on the TSS team jeopardized data acquisition, because of concern about her having access to those data. In honestly presenting their difficulties in engaging those who most suffer from racism and division in their Community Conversations, chapter 3's authors identify a challenge that can result from both internal and external factors—the challenge of fully realizing one's vision of ICEnR. Failure to acknowledge that challenge can even be a source of harm by making it seem as if inclusion, power sharing, or increased validity have been achieved fully when they have not.

The case studies presented here suggest the importance of intentionality in lessening and confronting these challenges and highlight a number of useful strategies. Faculty at the Duke School of Nursing have addressed conflicting expectations and norms on the part of students and community through preparatory student training, and cemented relationships with community partners by showing up at partners' events even outside of normal work hours. Mugoya and colleagues describe the Innovate with C.A.R.E. profile, which identifies each team member's role preference and provides information on how those preferences shape thoughts and behavior. Using this profile as they formed their partnership helped the Alabama team to increase the benefit they derived from their complementary differences and preempted some conflict. The team was also proactive in training peer leaders so that they could effectively collaborate on research. The TSS team delineates in chapter 4 a number of strategies that helped them partner effectively, including identifying beliefs, priorities, risks, and group norms as the group was forming; and shaping the roles of individual team members in response to external realities. They also note that the funding RWJF provided to their community team member was critical for her participation. Grover and Hines, in chapter 3, recommend use of the Restorative Justice Institute's approach to conversation and encounter among different members of a community, including the elements of meeting, narrative, emotion, understanding, and agreement.

The Utah team in chapter 7 was helped in meeting the community's tight deadlines by the flexibility of their home institution. They also accelerated their work through thoughtful division of labor and extensive use of student assistance (which had the added benefit of training the next generation of practitioners of community engagement, as does the Duke School of Nursing's collaboration with public housing sites). The Memphis team argues in chapter 5 that health impact assessment is a particularly good framework for supporting interdisciplinary, community-engaged, and translational work. They also describe identifying their knowledge gaps in public health early on and purposefully bringing on team members who filled those gaps. Finally, they used a number of strategies to forge common understandings among team members that allowed the team to collaborate effectively and set the stage for research translation. These included collective process mapping, identification and explication of terms and concepts that are different across sectors, targeted training (on local land-use regulation for the public health practitioners and epidemiology for the housing experts), and inclusion of partners who could play critical roles in collaboration, data collection and analysis, and translation. They also note the importance of the support provided by RWJF, specifically the training provided on policy change, communication, and outreach.

The variation in how ICEnR is "done" in this volume indicates that this approach is itself an important subject for research and scholarship. In fact, there is a growing body of literature on both the outcomes of engaged research (Harris et al., 2018; Oeztel et al., 2018; Staley, 2009; Viswanathan et al., 2004) and its practice (Eder et al., 2018; Oetzel et al., 2018). The imperative for ongoing inquiry into and dialogue about ICEnR stems from its goal of social change. For example, although—or, more likely, because—the authors of the case studies in this volume are highly attuned to the larger social structures and systems that contribute to poor health outcomes, they prioritize practicality. The Alabama team, for example, is thinking about how religion—a powerful force in the South that has contributed to the stigma around HIV—can become a vehicle for positive change. The Baton Rouge team, while pointing out that change must happen at both the community and individual levels, argues for starting work like theirs with the components of trauma-informed practice that are feasible to address within the given social and political environment, and embracing the potential of compromise to allow for progress. Such determinations raise important questions—ripe for additional empirical inquiry—about the strengths and weaknesses of different approaches to engaged research and translation. As a starting point, we offer some research questions suggested by the case studies in this volume, some of which are beginning to be addressed in the burgeoning body of work in this field, and some of which are newer. We have divided these questions into two categories: questions about effective approaches to ICEnR and questions about the outcomes of ICEnR.

Questions about effective approaches to ICEnR:

1. What are effective approaches to preparing members of affected communities to participate in ICEnR? How do we ask and enable the most marginalized to participate?

2. What are effective approaches to helping members of ICEnR teams understand and benefit from their differences? How do members of ICEnR teams create a foundation for successful collaboration?

3. Under what conditions are small wins transformed into a platform for more challenging endeavors? Under what conditions do small wins become a dead-end?

4. How do we effectively bring learners into the delicate endeavor of community engagement so as to facilitate this work and train the next generation of practitioners?

Questions about the outcomes of ICEnR efforts to promote social change

1. How can the powerful beliefs and institutions that fuel adverse cultural conditions for health (such as the stigma of HIV in the faith community) be transformed to support health?

2. How do the structures and processes of health impact assessment affect the outcomes of ICEnR, both in terms of policy change and change in the perspectives and knowledge of team members?

3.   What is the impact of exposure to community members' ideas about health on the thinking and behavior of policymakers, both elected and not elected?

4.   How does inclusion of service providers and policy advocates in ICEnR affect their work?

5.   What is gained and lost in terms of community, systems, and policy change as one moves up and down the spectrum from pragmatic action research to ICEnR rooted in liberation traditions?

6.   What types of messengers and what types of messages help to convince decision-makers in the healthcare policy and service delivery sectors to invest financially in housing as a SDoH?

The authors represented in this volume hope that our case studies and our reflections on them inspire others to engage with ICenR; afford them useful tools, frameworks, and examples for their endeavors; and provide inspiration and fodder for additional systematic inquiry on the practices and outcomes of this work. The most important message of this volume is that there is much to be gained by entering the intersections described here—the intersection between health and SDoH, the intersection between research knowledge and lived knowledge, the intersection between research and action. ICEnR is built on the belief that conversation and collaboration at these intersections matters. We hope that this volume contributes to that work.

References

Eder, M., Evans, E., Funes, M., Hong, H., Reuter, K., Ahmed, S., Calhoun, K., Corbie-Smith, G., Dave, G., DeFino, M., Harwood, E., Kissack, A., Kleinman, L. C., & Wallerstein, N. (2018). Defining and measuring community engagement and community-engaged research: CTSA community practices. *Progress in Community Health Partnerships Research Education and Action, 12*(2), 145–156.

Harris, J., Cook, T., Gibbs, L., Oeztel, J., Salsberg, J., Shinn, C., Springett, J., Wallerstein, N., & Wright, M. (2018). Searching for the impact of participation in health and health research: Challenges and methods. *BioMed Research International, 2018.* http://dx.doi.org/10.1155/2018/9427452

Oeztel, J. G., Wallerstein, N., Duran, B., Sanchez-Youngman, S., Nguyen, T., Woo, K., Wang, J., Schulz, A., Kaholokula, J. K., Israel, B., & Alegria, M. (2018). Impact of participatory health research: A test of the community-based participatory research conceptual model. *BioMed Research International, 2018.* http://dx.doi.org/10.1155/2018/7281405

Papinacolas, I., Woskie, L. R., & Jha, A. K. (2018). Health care spending in the United States and other high-income countries. *Journal of the American Medical Association, 319*(10), 1024–39.

Staley, K. (2009). *Exploring impact: Public involvement in NHS, public health, and social care research.* National Institutes for Health Research. Retrieved August 2, 2021, from http://www.invo.org.uk/posttypepublication/exploring-impact-public-involvement-in-nhs-public-health-and-social-care-research/

Viswanathan, M., Ammerman, A., Eng, E., Garlehner G., Lohr, K. N., Griffith, D., Rhodes, S., Samuel-Hodge, C., Mety, M., Lux, L., Webb, L., Sutton, S. F., Swinson, T., Jackman, A., & Whitener, L. (2004). Community-based participatory research: Assessing the evidence. *Evidence Report Technology Assessment (Suppl.)*(99), 1–8.

Wallerstein, N., & Duran, B. (2017). Theoretical, historical, and practice roots of CBPR. In N. Wallerstein, B. Duran, J. G. Oetzel, & M. Minkler (Eds.), *Community-based participatory research for health: Advancing social and health equity* (3rd ed.) (17–30). Jossey-Bass.

Bios

Editor Bio

Mina Silberberg, PhD, is an associate professor in the Duke Department of Family Medicine and Community Health and Vice-Chief for Research and Evaluation in the Division of Community Health. She also has faculty appointments at the Duke Global Health Institute and the Duke-Margolis Center for Health Policy and serves as the Director of the Community Engaged Research Initiative at the Duke Clinical and Translational Science Institute. Silberberg has been conducting community-engaged program evaluation, research, and policy analysis using mixed methods for more than two decades. She served as an editor and writer for the 2nd edition of the Principles of Community Engagement and is currently a member of the team authoring the 3rd edition. Her work has primarily focused on initiatives designed to address the health needs of low-income populations, and she has a particular interest in mobilization of multi-sectoral partnerships to address social drivers of health. Silberberg was a member of the first cohort (2016–2019) of the Interdisciplinary Research Fellows Program funded by the Robert Wood Johnson Foundation. Prior to coming to Duke, she was a senior policy analyst at the Rutgers Center for State Health Policy. Silberberg received her doctorate in political science from the University of California at Berkeley and completed postdoctoral training funded by NIA at the University of California at San Francisco.

Contributor Bios

Steve Barlow, JD, MA, co-founded Neighborhood Preservation, Inc., in Memphis, Tennessee. He directs community building and legislative advocacy initiatives and co-directs a legal clinic. He is an alumnus of the Robert Wood Johnson Interdisciplinary Research Leaders fellowship program.

Donna J. Biederman, DrPH, MN, RN, CPH, FAAN, is a faculty member at the Duke University School of Nursing where she directs the DUSON Community Health Improvement Partnership Program (D-CHIPP) and is also co-founder of the Durham Homeless Care Transitions program.

Emily Carmody, LCSW, is a leader to end homelessness. Emily was a case manager in shelters and outreach programs, and over the last decade, she has worked with the NC Coalition to End Homelessness to partner with communities across the state to design and implement systems that house people as quickly as possible. Emily is the co-creator of the Redesign Collaborative, LLC.

Shameka L. Cody, PhD, AGNP-C, is an assistant professor in the Capstone College of Nursing at the University of Alabama and a board-certified Adult-Gerontology Nurse Practitioner. Her research focuses on sleep and health disparities among older adults with HIV. She is well-funded and has 20+ publications in the field of HIV and cognitive aging.

Irene C. Felsman, DNP, MPH, RN, C-GH, has expertise in global community health and public health with an emphasis on community engagement methods and the development of culturally aligned interventions to improve health and access to care for women and children in diverse settings.

Laura Fish, PhD, MPH, is a behavioral scientist in the Department of Family Medicine and Community Health at Duke University and the Director of the Duke Cancer Institute Behavioral Health and Survey Research Core. Her research focuses on smoking cessation among vulnerable populations.

Pamela Foster, MD, MPH, is a professor in Community Medicine and Population Health and the Deputy Director of the Institute for Rural Health Research at the University of Alabama College of Community Health Sciences. A Preventive Medicine and Public Health physician, she specializes in health equity and community-engaged research.

Safiya George, PhD APRN-BC, FNAP, FAANP, is currently Dean and a professor at the Christine E. Lynn College of Nursing at Florida Atlantic University. She is a board-certified Adult Nurse Practitioner, a Distinguished Fellow of the National Academies of Practice, and a Fellow of the American Academy of Nurse Practitioners.

Leslie T. Grover, PhD, is an author and founder of the nonprofit research organization Assisi House, Inc. She helps communities achieve more equitable public policy outcomes. Her work centers the voices of the vulnerable through social justice art.

A. Michelle Hartman, DNP, RN, CPNP, has 23 years of nursing experience working with the pediatric population in acute, community, and global health settings. For the last 12 years she has taught undergraduate and graduate students with a special focus on community and global health.

Reva Hines, PhD, MPA, is an Alphonse Jackson Professor of Political Science at Southern University, Baton Rouge. She is an Interdisciplinary Research Leaders Cohort I Alumna. She is keenly interested in utilizing storytelling as a tool of empowerment and resiliency among marginalized groups.

Tammy Jacobs is the Educational Program Manager in the Resident Services Division with the City of Durham Housing Authority. Her mission has been to connect residents with local opportunities for success through continuous education, employment opportunities and resources. She has been with the Authority for over 10 years.

Billy Kirkpatrick, PhD is the Chief Executive Officer of Five Horizons Health Services, a nonprofit community-based organization that provides medical care, prevention education, supportive services, research, and advocacy to vulnerable populations in western Alabama and eastern Mississippi.

Heather Mountz, MPH, CPH, is a graduate from UNC-Chapel Hill's Gillings School of Public Health where she received a master's degree in Public Health Leadership. She is board-certified in Public Health by the National Board of Public Health Examiners.

George C. T. Mugoya, PhD, MPH, CRC, is an associate professor of Rehabilitation at the University of Alabama. His areas of academic, research, and clinical interest include improvement of the quality of life for individuals with chronic illness and disabilities including those with HIV/AIDS, substance abuse disorders, and mental health issues.

Devon Noonan, PhD, MPH, FNP-BC, is a nurse scientist and an associate professor in the Duke School of Nursing. Dr. Noonan's research is focused on using community-engaged approaches to develop health behavior change interventions with the goal of reducing risk for chronic disease.

Natalie Rich, MPH, currently works as the Region 5 Tobacco Prevention Manager for the Durham County Department of Public Health, overseeing tobacco policy and programs in eight counties in North Carolina. She received her BA and Master of Public Health degrees from UNC-Chapel Hill.

Joseph Schilling, LLM, JD, is a senior research associate in the Metropolitan Housing and Communities Policy Center and Research to Action Lab at the Urban Institute. He is an alumnus of the Interdisciplinary Research Leaders program led by the University of Minnesota with support from the Robert Wood Johnson Foundation.

Christina Plerhoples Stacy, PhD, is a principal research associate in the Metropolitan Housing and Communities Policy Center at the Urban Institute, where she specializes in urban economics, equity, and inclusion. Her work focuses on the intersection of economics and urban spaces and how housing, transportation, local economies, health, and crime interact.

Lina Svedin, PhD, is an associate professor of Political Science at the University of Utah where she teaches courses in public administration and public policy in the Programs of Public Affairs. Her research spans diverse policy topics, ethics, risk, and crisis management.

Jesús Valero, PhD, is an assistant professor in the Department of Political Science at the University of Utah where he teaches courses on public and nonprofit management. Jesús' research explores government-nonprofit partnerships and effective leadership in nonprofit organizations.

Acknowledgments

The reviewers of this book and its individual chapters challenged the authors to think more deeply about our experiences and what could be learned from them. We offer our thanks to these insightful individuals: Jefferey Donnithorne, Sheri Johnson, David Levine, Kermit Lind, Kristy Lowenthal, James E. McLean, Yeeli Mui, Nicole Prewitt, Albert Samuels, and Steven Smith. Additional thanks for the many ways—both intellectual and pragmatic—in which the series editors, Farrah Jacquez and Lina Svedin, made this book possible. Sarah Muncy, Alexandra Nash, and Elizabeth Scarpelli shepherded us patiently through the publication process. They and others at University of Cincinnati Press brought their considerable expertise to the production of this volume, as did Marilyn Campbell and Kathie Klee.

We are also grateful for the support of the Robert Wood Johnson Foundation through its Interdisciplinary Research Leaders (IRL) program, which funded much of the work described in this volume and brought the authors together. We owe a further debt of gratitude to the IRL national program office out of the University of Minnesota for the many ways in which the office's faculty, staff, and community leaders enriched our work. Finally, we are grateful to the family, friends, teachers, and colleagues who have supported us throughout the journeys from which this book comes.

Index

n = footnote; *t* = table